Loneliness Among Children With Special Needs

Malka Margalit

Loneliness Among Children With Special Needs

Theory, Research, Coping, and Intervention

Springer-Verlag
New York Berlin Heidelberg London Paris
Tokyo Hong Kong Barcelona Budapest

Malka Margalit
Department of Educational Sciences
School of Education
Faculty of Humanities
Tel Aviv University
Ramat Aviv, 69978
Israel

With 6 figures.

Library of Congress Cataloging-in-Publication Data
Margalit, Malka.
Loneliness among children with special needs : theory, research, coping, and intervention / Malka Margalit.
p. cm.
Includes bibliographical references and index.
ISBN-13:978-1-4612-7611-1
1. Loneliness in children. 2. Learning disabled children --Psychology. 3. Developmentally disabled children--Psychology.
I. Title.
BF723.L64M37 1994
155.45'2--dc20 93-32707

Printed on acid-free paper.

Softcover reprint of the hardcover 1st edition 1994

Production managed by Jim Harbison; manufacturing supervised by Jacqui Ashri.
Camera-ready copy provided by the author.

9 8 7 6 5 4 3 2 1

ISBN-13:978-1-4612-7611-1 e-ISBN-13:978-1-4612-2622-2
DOI: 10.1007/978-1-4612-2622-2

to my husband

Preface

The field of loneliness has been characterized by a diversity and richness of perspectives. There is also a shared view, often based on clinical experience and research outcomes, that children with disabilities experience more loneliness than nondisabled children. It is surprising that regardless of the extensive research already in existence that focuses on the social deficiencies of these children and their relations to social, cognitive, and affective processes, efforts have not been directed toward clarifying loneliness and its implications.

This book was designed to integrate the existing knowledge, research, and applications in order to offer a model for understanding the loneliness experiences of these children. It is based on research that was conducted at Tel Aviv University by the special education research team including graduate students who were intrigued by this subject. The disabilities manifested by the children in this volume can be denoted as mild disabilities—such as learning disabilities, mild mental retardation, behavior disorders, and emotional difficulties—that interfered with age-appropriate functioning and adjustment and created the need for these children to receive special education services.

The book is divided into five major sections. In the first section, loneliness is presented as an aspect of personality, in an attempt to clarify the various conceptual approaches and to discuss the characteristics of the lonely child. The second section is devoted to environments and interpersonal relations, with an emphasis on home and peer relations. The third section is concerned with the subtyping of loneliness and adjustment, leading to the identification of four subgroups of children with disabilities. In the fourth section, the outcomes of loneliness through coping and interventions are discussed. Finally, the last section provides a summary of research using the proposed loneliness model for children with disabilities.

Feeling lonely suggests a passive orientation—the disabled child expresses dissatisfaction through passive helplessness. Coping with loneliness suggests an active approach aiming to enhance a change in behavior and feelings. I hope that this volume will prove useful to researchers, clinicians, educators, and other professionals who see the importance of companionship for promoting growth of children with special needs, and the costs of loneliness for current life quality and future adjustment.

MALKA MARGALIT

Acknowledgments

I would like to express my appreciation to a number of people who encouraged and assisted me in my efforts to prepare this book. The case study descriptions presented in this volume emerged through my work on the Special Education Technology Project at Tel Aviv University. I wish to thank Yad-Avi-HaYishuv for their continuous help and support in this project. Special thanks go to Michal Al-Yagon for her devoted work in directing the project, counseling the teachers, and collecting research data; and to Meira Efrati who worked dedicatedly with her, providing her unique perspective of the subject. I would also like to express my gratitude to the editorial assistance provided by Dee B. Ankonina, who spent many hours reviewing the manuscript. Thanks are extended as well to my graduate students and especially to Zohar Dayan for her technical assistance. Finally, to the children who have disabilities, and to their teachers and parents, I voice my deepest gratitude, for having shared their feelings of loneliness in order to help develop a better understanding of these experiences that may improve the life quality of children with special needs.

Contents

Section III. A Subtyping Approach

Section IV. Coping and Intervention

Section V. Epilogue: Development, Disabilities, and Loneliness

Section I
Loneliness Attributes

1 Theoretical Approaches to Loneliness

Psychologists, sociologists, and anthropologists all concur in their regard of humans as social beings who require the support and companionship of other individuals throughout different stages of the life cycle. Any understanding of human existence must clarify people's need for interpersonal interactions and must explore the emergence of connections and companionship (Storr, 1988). People may characterize their relationships along a continuum consisting of several measures such as good or bad, close or distant, intensive or superficial, fulfilling or frustrating. Loneliness represents a person's sense of inner dissatisfaction in contrast to a desired quality and quantity of interpersonal relationships (Spitzberg & Hurt, 1987). In order to establish an in-depth evaluation of connectedness, loneliness, and social distress, the richness of human relations should be fully acknowledged, exploring the role of these relations in promoting a sense of personal coherence.

All people, regardless of age or sex, experience loneliness at some time in their lives, but some do so much more than others. For most people, intense feelings of loneliness are short lived. For others, loneliness and social alienation are persistent realities of everyday experience. Poets and philosophers have debated the existential meaning of loneliness, while researchers have attempted to clarify why some individuals endure the experience of loneliness more than do others despite access to seemingly comparable objective social networks. Other areas of empirical inquiry include such questions as which situations are more conducive to experiencing loneliness, why some people seem to cope with it more effectively, and at what age stages such feelings predominate. Human beings spend a significant amount of time alone, yet solitude is not always perceived as distressing or as arousing feelings of loneliness and isolation.

The fact that loneliness has been found to predict feelings of hopelessness and depressed mood even in the early stages of development (Page, 1991b) emphasizes the importance of early identification and intervention programs for loneliness in order to prevent a later sense of despair and its consequences upon emotional health, adjustment, and development. A rapidly growing trend in social research is currently targeting children, with a focus on youngsters who lack friends or feel lonely and isolated in school. Much of the increased research interest stems from evidence indicating that children who experience poor peer relations and social alienation constitute "at risk" populations who may demonstrate both reduced opportunities for social learning and greater adjustment problems during adulthood (Asher, Parkhurst, Hymel, & Williams, 1990; Luftig, 1987).

A vast body of research has already documented the social difficulties and peer rejection manifested by children who have cognitive and emotional disorders, clearly positioning these children within the boundaries of the population defined as "at risk" for later social maladjustment. The social alienation of students with learning disabilities, mental retardation, and behavior disorders can easily be expected to be linked to a greater sense of loneliness among these youngsters in comparison to their peers. Yet, despite their expected intensified distress, little investigation has centered on the subjective loneliness experiences of these young people who have disabilities.

The study of loneliness among children with disabilities is in fact the study of children's social connections and interrelations, in all their subtlety and variability, as related to the study of the self, in terms of how the children view themselves, how others view them, and how they feel about these perceptions and conceptions by others. This exploration of children's perceptions, conceptions, and feelings may provide valuable information not only on the individual children but also on the social climate in their inherent social institutions and natural systems such as schools and families, thus pinpointing breakdowns in social interactions that reflect systemic difficulties originating from a mismatch between students and their environments (Peplau & Perlman, 1982).

This book represents an effort to integrate empirical research and theoretical conceptualization, in order to elucidate the multidimensional construct of loneliness among students with special needs, with an emphasis on affective, cognitive, and behavioral aspects. Several questions will be discussed, such as How can loneliness be defined? What types of situations and what kinds of personal characteristics may trigger the loneliness experience of these youngsters? What factors can mediate or buffer these personal characteristics and situational variables? This direction of study on loneliness aims to enhance our awareness of the current life quality among students with disabilities, to facilitate the prediction of future difficulties in adjustment, highlighting their social context, and to point out directions for intervention. The present chapter will first provide a brief overview of the theoretical definitions of loneliness as a multidimensional construct, and then will touch upon the developmental and contextual frameworks necessary for its exploration in terms of children with disabilities.

What is loneliness?

The variability in definitions of loneliness seems to reflect differences in envisioning the nature of the social deficiency experienced by lonely individuals within their environments. Woodward's (1988, p. 4) definition attempted to provide a comprehensive description of the construct, avoiding causal models: "Loneliness is a feeling of being alone and disconnected or alienated from positive people, places and things."

Peplau and Perlman (1982) proposed three main theoretical approaches to the understanding of the concept:

1 Human needs approach
2 Cognitive process approach
3 Behavioral approach

Human needs approach

The human needs approach (Fromm-Reichman, 1959; Sullivan, 1953) viewed loneliness within a developmental context, as related to unfulfilled individual needs for various types of social interrelations at different stages of development. Within this approach, the unfulfilled developmental need is posited as constituting the cause for later interpersonal difficulties. Sullivan (1953) described loneliness as the unpleasant experience related to the inadequate discharge of the need for human intimacy or for close interpersonal relations. Similarly, Weiss (1973) described that loneliness is caused not by being alone, but by being without some definite needed relationship, or as a response to the absence of a specific relational provision.

For children with disabilities, this approach pinpoints their atypical development as the root of their increased loneliness experience and focuses attention on family relations and the parents' coping with their disabled children. The needs of these children for intimate, supportive relations may be increased due to their greater experience of failure and frustration. However, adults' and peers' abilities to meet these needs in the environment will be affected by their own distress and reactions to the disabilities (Margalit, 1990a).

Research within this orientation has directed interest toward the subjective aspects of social needs and interrelations throughout development, from the infant's early striving for intimate interrelations, through the young child's attempts to achieve a sense of belonging to a group of peers, and onward to the adolescent's and adult's search for assurance of being acknowledged and appreciated by a significant group of valued persons. When children experience difficulties due to their increased needs for support and help, or when adults and peers reveal failures or difficulties in meeting these needs, the loneliness experience may be considered as related to these unfulfilled human needs.

Cognitive approach

The cognitive process approach underscores perceptions, comparisons, and evaluations of social relations. Peplau and Perlman (1982) proposed that loneliness occurs when the individual perceives a discrepancy between two factors: the desired and the achieved pattern of social relations. The comparison between the actual and the desired quality and quantity of social relations is usually related to the comparison of self-perceptions and perceptions of others. According to this approach, such a comparison may lead to the experience of loneliness -- when actual relations are seen as fewer than desired and as superficial in quality -- or to the experience of "invasion of privacy" -- when actual relations are seen as too intimate and as larger and closer than desired (Altman, 1975). More than nondisabled children, children with disabilities may experience not only different types of initial cognitive difficulties that affect their social reality testing, but also a range of secondary subjective perceptions and attributional trends that reflect their long history of failure and frustrations. Cognitive cues regarding social dissatisfaction revolve around the theme of wanting a type of social relationship that is currently lacking, such as more frequent interrelations, a wider social network, and/or more intimate or closer relationships (Peplau, Miceli, & Morasch, 1982). Underlying these cues is the belief that a change in social relations will affect the person's feelings of distress.

Research within this orientation has focused not on the need fulfillment but rather on cognitive processes that predict loneliness and on the attributions provided for the explanation of isolation and social rejection. Cognitive models utilize subjective perceptions and standards, wherein loneliness indicates the subjective dissatisfaction with one's social relations with peers and adults. Within this model, the experience of loneliness is measured not by objective indices of the person's actual social relations, with measures such as the number of friends and the size of the social network, but rather by the perceived discrepancy between reality and the desired pattern or qualitative standard for these relations. Two children may have similar patterns of interpersonal relations, yet one is content whereas the other experiences loneliness. Children identify themselves as lonely individuals following an inferential process, in which they map out their private experiences within a more general social map (Peplau, Miceli, & Morasch, 1982). An important question in exploring disabled children's sense of social isolation lies not only in their self-perceptions and attributions but also in determining how they select their group of reference for the inferential process: Do lonely children feel dissatisfied in their social relations with other disabled children like themselves, or does loneliness reflect their desire for relations with their nondisabled peers, or both?

Behavioral approach

A behavioral approach conceptualizes insufficient social reinforcements as the source of loneliness feelings. According to this approach, social relationships can be treated as a particular class of reinforcement, and loneliness can be viewed in part as a response to the absence or insufficient amount of important social reinforcements (Young, 1982). The learning experience of socialization, according to the behavioral approach, is thus directly related to a reinforcement framework within the child's environment. The quantity and quality of interpersonal contacts that the person finds satisfying and reinforcing is viewed as the product of his/her reinforcement history. Children with disabilities are seen as experiencing more aversive social relations, originating in biased perceptions from their potential social partners and in less satisfactory interpersonal contacts. In different contextual conditions, these children miss out on the reinforcing forces such as positive affect related to successful attempts to initiate close relations with peers and adults, leading to predominantly negative and frustrating social experiences. According to this orientation, loneliness is also defined in part by the presence of some negative aversive emotions that are a function of the attributions made by the individual to explain the dissatisfying social interrelations and personal frustrations (Young, 1982).

Shared loneliness concepts

Regardless of the different emphases within these three approaches toward defining loneliness, several areas of agreement can be detected (Russell, Cutrona, Rose, & Yurko, 1984):

Loneliness is an aversive experience. Similar to other negative affective states such as anxiety or depression, loneliness is an unpleasant and distressing experience. Although loneliness has not been shown to be related to one unique set of emotions, sadness, pain, and unhappiness are the accompanying feelings most frequently mentioned. Lonely children describe their unhappy moods using sentences such as "I am sad" or "I feel sorry for myself," and they depict themselves as feeling bored and depressed.

Loneliness is a subjective experience. As a subjective experience, loneliness may be related or unrelated to the objectively measured existing social network. Children can feel lonely even while in a group, or, alternatively, may remain alone but feel content and not lonely. In expressing a feeling of loneliness, children evaluate themselves using only subjective social comparisons (i.e., perceptions of other individuals) as a criterion. For instance, children may say that everybody else has fun except for them, or that all of the other children they know have many good friends while they remain alone and feel lonely. The consideration of the loneliness construct as a subjective experience has been supported by the lack of distinct relations between observed social interrelations, sociometric status ratings, and reported loneliness feelings, and by the insufficient covariance between reported loneliness feelings and the individual's amount of social contacts (Rook, 1984).

The only reliable report for loneliness feelings can be achieved through the individual's own self-report. Weiss (1982, 1987) stated that in loneliness research no objective correlate exists to indicate if loneliness is present without having to ask. In view of the fact that self-reports are the only reliable sources tapping children's loneliness experiences, research (Asher, Parkhurst, Hymel, & Williams, 1990; Luftig, 1987) has attempted to assess loneliness in relation to estimated social competence, and to identify whether sensitivity to the reality of one's loneliness is related to factors in normative and atypical development. Results confirmed that children understand what the loneliness construct means and that even young preschool (Cassidy & Asher, 1992) and/or disabled children such as students with learning disabilities (Margalit & Al-Yagon, in press) can report their subjective experiences.

Loneliness is distinct from solitude. Loneliness, reflecting the individual's subjective perception of his/her deficiencies within the network of social relations, is distinct from aloneness, which indicates a tangible situation. The subjective deficiencies may be evaluated quantitatively (i.e., inadequate size of the social network) or qualitatively (i.e., lack of intimacy with others). Solitude, being different from loneliness, involves a deliberate choice to be alone. The motivation for solitude may stem from a wish for reflection, meditation, or some purposeful activity such as studying or pursuing an interest or hobby. In contrast to the consistently negative affect related to loneliness, solitude can be viewed as a pleasant, positive, and sometimes even desirable situation that may promote a creative experience or provide an opportunity for rest from stressful reality and overwork (Marcoen & Goossens, 1990).

Types of loneliness

A survey of research reveals the existing theoretical disagreement concerning the structure of the loneliness construct (Russell, Cutrona, Rose, & Yurko, 1984). The traditional approach (Andersson, 1985; Andersson, Mullins & Johnson, 1987; Weiss, 1982) views loneliness as consisting of two distinct components: (a) emotional loneliness and (b) social loneliness (Weiss, 1973, 1974). Emotional loneliness can be seen as the unsatisfied need for intimacy and close social contact (e.g., having a good friend), whereas social loneliness can be viewed as the absence of a place in the accepting community (e.g., belonging to a network of friends). According to the traditional orientation, the same word "loneliness" may be used by various people to represent distinct subjective experiences and meanings.

The second approach considers the loneliness construct to represent a common core of experience regardless of age, sex, or cultural conditions (Hojat, 1982b). According to this approach, although different people may emphasize various aspects of their private experience of social and emotional isolation, the construct's components are viewed as clearly interrelated rather than as distinct experiences.

Emotional loneliness

The emotional loneliness dimension refers to a deficiency in socio-emotional bonding and intimate relations with another person and can be seen as leading to feelings of anxiety and isolation (Weiss, 1973). Persons may feel lonely in the sense of being emotionally isolated regardless of whether or not they are involved with others. This type of loneliness has been found to be best predicted by the absence of an early attachment figure in one's life. In light of the assumption that this problem stems from a deficit in the individual's capacity for interpersonal bonding, treatment should accentuate basic personality patterns that may well have had their origins in the family orientation during socialization processes early in life. The promotion of new intimate relationships that provide a sense of attachment has been proposed as the "cure" or remediation for a sense of emotional loneliness. The introduction of any change into an individual's interpersonal functioning presumes an emotional or psychological capacity for socio-emotional bonding.

Social loneliness

Social loneliness, referring to the lack of a recognized social role and the lack of a network of social relationships, can be characterized by feelings of boredom, aimlessness, and depression (Weiss, 1973). The socially lonely individual seeks participation in activities within networks or groups that will accept him or her as a member. This type of loneliness was best predicted by a lack of reassurance of personal worth and identity in a group. Intentional exclusion and rejection by a group of individuals who share common interests may prevent gratifications and rewards that can only be mediated by social interchange. Remediation here should target the individual's social role, entry into a network of friendships, and the sense of belonging to a group or social network. Engagement in social activities and enhancement of feelings of belonging, whether based on shared concerns, interests, work, or other activities, may alleviate the feelings of social loneliness and reinforce a reassurance of one's own worth.

Interrelations between the loneliness types

Hojat (1982a) supported the distinction between social and emotional isolation, highlighting the multivariate nature of loneliness feelings. She found that individuals who reported that their parents had not devoted enough time to them and did not understand them, felt lonely. Those who recounted that they did not get along with their peers in childhood, also tended to experience more loneliness. Her research study exemplified that individuals who feel lonely tend to use the same concept of "loneliness" to express different contents and to describe a different pattern and structure of self-perceptions.

Russell, Cutrona, Rose, and Yurko's (1984) research also provided partial support for Weiss' (1973) differentiation. Their study indicated that social and emotional loneliness are distinct experiential states, yet they share a high degree of associated common experience. Both social and emotional isolation were consistently found to be positively related to the quality and quantity of friendships, suggesting the varied functions of friendships for the individual throughout development. Depression was also related to both emotional and social isolation (although the relation was stronger with emotional isolation), whereas anxiety was found to be related only to social isolation.

The ability to distinguish between aspects of one's loneliness experience may be connected to age-related capacities, suggesting the central significance of a developmental perspective for its conceptualization.

The developmental perspective

Research focusing on the etiology of subjective loneliness feelings has emphasized the importance of the developmental perspective for a full understanding of the loneliness construct (Andersson, 1986; Andersson, Mullins, & Johnson, 1987). Asher's research substantiated the viability of this direction of study by demonstrating that children as young as the preschool age already have fairly well-developed concepts of loneliness (Asher, Parkhurst, Hymel, & Williams, 1990; Cassidy & Asher, 1992). The developmental perspective appears to hold special importance for students with disabilities, whose developmental course is inherently characterized by difficulties, failures, and frustrations that are likely to increase these youngsters' risk of experiencing such feelings. Within the developmental construct, two distinct classes of causes for loneliness may be identified (Rothbaum & Weisz, 1989):

Precipitators. Events leading to changes in actual social relations such as entering into a new school, moving into a new neighborhood, or being in places where it is difficult to meet new people can precipitate the onset of the experience of loneliness. Developmental changes in the child's capacity, desire, or need for social relations during the life cycle may initiate a sense of loneliness if they are not accompanied by corresponding changes in actual relations.

Predisposers. When changes and life transitions occur, certain factors may predispose individuals to become lonely or to persist in remaining lonely over time. At each stage of

> development, children are predisposed to certain kinds of problems and are protected from others because of their developing abilities, beliefs about their power, and their desire or motivation for control. Their sense of control over life events bridges between considerations of a cognitive-developmental and of a motivational nature (Rothbaum & Weisz, 1989).

Cognitive development can be conceptualized as one of the factors making the child susceptible to certain problems rather than as causing those problems (Rothbaum & Weisz, 1989). Its impact may be viewed as a predisposer, setting the stage for the problems more or less likely to appear at particular ages. However, cognitive development alone does not determine whether a problem will arise. Specific problems reflect specific beliefs (e.g., helplessness reflects low attributions of one's ability), and the level of cognitive functioning is only one of the factors predisposing these beliefs. A variety of personal and situational variables predict the child's initial vulnerability to experiencing loneliness. Yet lonely children, once being predisposed to loneliness, also find it more difficult to further establish satisfying social relations. Thus, a child who has deficient social skills may find it difficult to develop or maintain satisfying relations, and these deficient skills may then be viewed as predispositional factors for later loneliness experiences.

It has not yet been clarified whether loneliness feelings can be best explained by precipitators such as a reaction to a current experience or a mismatch between a child's abilities and his or her environment's expectations, or by predisposers such as a vulnerability factor having its roots in early childhood and emerging when combined with stress and other variables.

Rubin and Mills (1988) linked the concept of social withdrawal with a developmental perspective, emphasizing the multidimensional, age-related nature of the construct. They found that some forms of withdrawal and solitude may be viewed as normative at certain ages, yet may reflect and predict disorders at other points in life. These researchers differentiated between two types of behavioral solitude: passive isolation and active isolation. Passive isolation usually involves quite constructive or exploratory behavior. During preschool, this behavior may reflect an interest in mastering nonsocial tasks through exploration and constructive play. During elementary-school years, when children spend most of their time in constructive activities (i.e., schoolwork), the child who continues to play alone may be reflecting social anxiety, peer rejection, and an increased risk for developing internalizing disorders such as anxiety, loneliness, and depression. The second form of withdrawal -- active isolation -- is characterized by cognitively immature behavior and may predict loneliness.

Inconsistent research findings for age differences have been revealed by reports of loneliness. For example, a consensus exists in the literature that adolescents' active search for identity, separation from parental dependence, and increased need for peer relations, would all be expected to result in greater loneliness. However, only some research has demonstrated the expected developmental increase in loneliness, whereas several other studies failed to reveal significant age differences at all, and still others pinpointed a higher incidence of loneliness among younger children with and without disabilities (Avrahami, 1992; Luftig, 1987; Margalit & Ronen, 1993; Zehavi, 1992).

The fact that some studies revealed more loneliness in younger groups of children may be explained in two ways: It may be that, in reality, the adolescents do experience higher levels of loneliness as earlier conceptualized, yet the younger children are more open in disclosing their inner feelings of loneliness than are their older counterparts and express it more fully. Alternatively, it may be assumed that younger children experience less freedom and mobility to form friendships outside of school. Thus, in-class rejection from peers may more directly affect their feelings of loneliness as measured in the school setting. The inconsistent results from these studies may also reflect sample differences, restricting our ability to make generalized conclusions as to the existence of significant developmental trends. In view of the cross-sectional methodology in the research literature, it appears that only comprehensive longitudinal studies that follow the developmental paths of different samples of children with and without disabilities may clarify the direction of the age-related development of loneliness experiences.

Gender perspectives

Similar inconsistencies were found in gender difference studies. Bell (1991) found in his research that male and female adults did not differ regarding their loneliness or levels of friendship network density, although females reported closer ties to their friends. Measures of density -- the extent to which one feels close to one's friends -- and of loneliness were negatively related, and individuals who felt more closely connected to their friends were less likely to experience loneliness. On the other hand, Medora and Woodward (1986) found that females in late adolescence tended to be lonelier than their male peers. Male and female children did not report different levels of loneliness experiences in samples of disabled and nondisabled children alike (Brennan, 1992; Efrati, 1993; Margalit, 1991a, 1991b, 1993a; Margalit & Ben-Dov, 1992; Margalit & Ronen, 1993). Marcoen and Goossens (1990) also did not find significant gender differences, with the exception of attitudes toward loneliness. Females reported a more negative view of loneliness. Similarly, Brennan (1982) did not find consistent sex differences, yet girls tended to agree more than boys with self-descriptions such as "I feel lonely." These inconsistent differences highlighted the need for detailed interviews and extensive research in order to clarify a gender-related conceptualization of loneliness and relationships (Maccoby, 1990).

Disabilities and loneliness

Loneliness experiences have often been linked with reported difficulties in peer relations (Asher, Parkhurst, Hymel, & Williams, 1990). Children who have the greatest difficulties with their peer relations, feeling rejected and alienated, are those who report the highest levels of loneliness. However, loneliness is not an uncommon experience among children. Significant loneliness is an experience reported by at least 10 to 15 percent of all students (Iverson & Eichler, 1992). Luftig (1987) found through analysis of single items on a loneliness questionnaire that 22% of second graders, 20% of fourth graders, and 12% of sixth graders indicated strong agreement with the statement "I feel alone." Similar proportions were found for items such as "I'm lonely" and "I don't have anyone to play with." It seems that a significant number of children feel lonely and isolated, according to measures that tapped loneliness feelings in school.

Children with disabilities have been considered to be less competent socially and more rejected by peers and thus can be expected to experience more loneliness than do nondisabled children. Only a few studies have provided comparisons between disabled and nondisabled children in these areas. In an investigation of loneliness feelings among 122 students with learning disabilities, in comparison to those of 120 nondisabled youngsters, the learning disabled students were found to be less socially accepted and more lonely than were their nondisabled peers (Margalit & Ben-Dov, 1992). Two additional studies (Unger, 1992; Zehavi, 1992) replicated these results, adding that sadness was the emotion most frequently related to loneliness, whereas anger and boredom were reported less often.

Similar findings have been shown for other disability groups. The loneliness feelings of 170 hearing impaired undergraduate students from eight mainstreamed colleges and universities were found to be higher than those of 230 hearing undergraduates (Murphy & Newlon, 1987), with no loneliness differences evidenced as a function of relative hearing loss severity or gender. These results were substantiated by Luftig's (1988) and Williams and Asher's (1990, 1992) studies reporting that many students with mental retardation experience loneliness. However, Williams and Asher's (1992) study pinpointed attention at the impact of gender as reflected in loneliness comparisons, with boys reporting more loneliness. The comparison of loneliness levels between three groups of disabled adolescents -- with mental retardation, learning disabilities, and behavior difficulties -- revealed that the group with mental retardation reported the highest levels of loneliness and that the group with learning disabilities felt less lonely than those with mental retardation and more lonely than those with behavior difficulties (Margalit, 1993b). In another study (Margalit, 1991a), no significant differences were reported between the loneliness levels of students with learning disabilities and students with behavior disorders, although the groups differed with regard to the relations they demonstrated between loneliness and aggressive or disruptive behavior. For the behavior disordered students, the more they evidenced disruptiveness, the less lonely they felt. For the children with learning disabilities, a positive relationship was found between loneliness and disruptive behavior, where higher aggressiveness was related to their increased loneliness.

Conclusions

Loneliness is affected by the match or mismatch between one's social needs, desires, or skills and the perceived realities of one's social environment. Primary factors may predispose children to the loneliness experience, and secondary self-related or situational variables may maintain or reinforce it. These factors may include the extent to which the child fails to develop meaningful relations, to bridge social or interpersonal space, and to cope with feelings of being alienated and different from others in their immediate social environment. The personal characteristics and handicapping conditions among children with disabilities may not only predispose them to loneliness, but also may render it more difficult for them to cope with feelings of loneliness, whether their dominant pattern reflects the social and/or the emotional components of isolation, when they arise.

The social situation of children with disabilities emphasizes the urgency of the need for concentrated research efforts to clarify the nature and causes of loneliness. The nature of the loneliness experience may be related to unique aspects of personality in terms of individualized needs, abilities, and developmental paths typified by deficits and failures. Thus, the study of loneliness among youngsters with disabilities calls for a careful examination not only of individual histories and characteristics that make these children vulnerable to experiencing extreme levels of loneliness and peer rejection, but also of the environmental features that initiate or maintain their feelings of exclusion and rejection.

The goals of this book are to examine in depth the loneliness experience reported by children with disabilities as related to their individual characteristics and social systems at home and at school. Loneliness of children with and without disabilities is a painful experience that may represent different content areas, but always signals the existence of a failure in the valued area of interpersonal relationships. In order to ensure a deeper understanding of the meaning of the loneliness experience, within the ecological paradigm, varied aspects of human connections within environments will be described. However, prior to the exploration of interpersonal relations in the family and peer settings, the personal factors characterizing lonely children will be the focus of discussion.

2 Personal Aspects of Loneliness

Much debate has been related to a major research question: Is loneliness an individual or an interpersonal problem? The extent to which the experience is a product of personal or interpersonal processes is still unclear, constituting a central issue for research. Several studies have conceptualized the manner and extent to which the loneliness experience can be viewed as a function of individual personality structure, reflecting levels of personal emotional adjustment and pinpointing social skill deficits (Goswick & Jones, 1981; Hojat, 1982b).

These subjective findings suggested that the experience of loneliness cannot be disconnected from its interpersonal or social context. However, loneliness is at least in part predicted by personal processes reflecting individual differences and unique personality characteristics. Observers have rated lonely individuals as significantly less interpersonally skilled, and children who were shown to be rejected by their peers according to sociometric assessments reported feeling more lonely than did their peers (Asher, Parkhurst, Hymel, & Williams, 1990). Thus, although loneliness may be viewed as a private psychological experience, it appears to manifest itself within an interpersonal reality.

In conclusion, it seems that both personality dispositions and social situations each contribute to the amount of loneliness an individual may experience (Cheek & Busch, 1981). In an attempt to clarify processes that lead to loneliness, this chapter will focus discussion on personality aspects such as attribution style, self-esteem, and social skills and will present the individual perspective through variables such as age and sex differences that may be considered to be related to loneliness. The contextual aspects of loneliness within different ecological conditions such as family, peer, and school environments will be explored in Chapters 3 and 4.

Within the group of theories highlighting the personality constructs related to loneliness, several traits have been consistently reported: shyness, withdrawal tendencies, anxiety in general and social anxiety in particular, dependence on others, negative self-concept, introverted character, poor social skills, and less willingness to take social risks (Kalliopuska & Laitinen, 1991; Overholser, 1992; Peplau & Perlman, 1982; Van-Buskirk & Duke, 1991). In particular, self-esteem, social skills, and attribution style were pinpointed as significant predictors of the loneliness experience (Inderbitzen-Pisaruk, Clark, & Solano, 1992).

Self-perceptions

The relations between loneliness and low self-esteem are considered reciprocal (Inderbitzen-Pisaruk, Clark, & Solano, 1992; Peplau, Miceli, & Morasch, 1982). Negative patterns of self-perceptions were found to be associated with loneliness among adults (Hymel, Frank, & Freigang, 1985; Short, Schatschneider, & Friebert, 1992). Lonely adults and children alike reported lower self-esteem than did their non-lonely peers. A poor sense of self-esteem may cause people to interpret social interactions in a negative way, and children who devaluate themselves have difficulty believing that their peers may see them differently. Lonely individuals often feel unloved and incompetent.

Among children who consistently fail academically due to their learning or behavior disabilities, many have been documented for their lower self-esteem (Margalit, Raviv, & Pahn-Steinmetz, 1988; Margalit & Zak, 1984; Rogers & Saklofske, 1985), poorer self-perceptions, and more negative feelings of overall self-worth (Bear, Clever, & Proctor, 1991; Margalit, 1985). Extended periods of loneliness may lower these children's self-esteem, and their lower self-esteem may then increase the children's loneliness, which in turn may further impede their sense of self-worth and efficacy. The disabilities factor in the children's functioning seems to add a third component that may further promote this reciprocal processing. Their loneliness may be interrelated not only to feelings of lower self-esteem but also to their realistic experience of failure in academic and social areas.

The concept of perceived self-efficacy within social cognitive theory (Bandura, 1988) provides a more explicit account of why children with disabilities may feel lonely and socially isolated. Perceived self-efficacy is concerned with children's beliefs in their capabilities to mobilize the motivation, cognitive resources, and courses of action needed to exercise control over given events (Ozer & Bandura, 1990). In line with Bandura's theories of the determinants and mechanisms of avoidant behavior (such as withdrawal and social isolation) that may lead to loneliness feelings, children with disabilities tend to appraise their social reality as uncontrolled, leading to rejection by peers, frustrations, and anxiety (Margalit, 1990a). Individuals' beliefs regarding their own efficacy influence the types of anticipatory scenarios that they construct and reiterate in their thinking. Those who judge themselves as less efficacious in many important age-related tasks are more inclined to visualize themselves as experiencing failure scenarios, and to dwell on how things will go wrong. Such thinking or ineffective beliefs weaken motivation and undermine performance (Bandura, 1989). Beliefs about self-efficacy affect the self-regulation of cognitive processes, increasing the feelings of hopelessness related to social alienation and decreasing motivation to change social relations. Those students who believe they cannot manage potential threats may experience high levels of anxiety arousal (Bandura, 1986) that are also associated with high social anxiety.

Social skills

Social skills are those socially accepted, learned behaviors that enable the individual to interact effectively with peers and to avoid socially unacceptable responses (Gresham, 1986; Gresham & Elliott, 1984). Erickson's (1968) outline of age-related tasks in psychosocial development underscored the importance of mastering age-related social skills that provide the foundation for satisfactory social interrelations during adolescence and adult life. Strategies for entering into groups, initiating interactions, sharing, helping, and requesting help are just some examples of social skills (Gresham & Elliott, 1987, 1990). It is not surprising that children who have disabilities that are rooted in ineffective learning processes have often been found to experience difficulties in acquiring age-appropriate social skills (Gresham & Reschly, 1986; Margalit, in press; Margalit &

Ben-Dov, 1992; Odom, McConnell, & McEvoy, 1992). These poorer social skills appear to be pervasive in school and home settings, consistent for both interpersonal and self-related behaviors, and stable across different judges such as teachers, parents, and peers.

Social skill deficits

Social skill deficits have been considered to be an important predictor of the loneliness experience for children with and without disabilities at different age levels (Inderbitzen-Pisaruk, Clark, & Solano, 1992). Negative correlations were consistently found between the loneliness experience and social skills ratings among children with mental retardation (Avrahami, 1992) and learning disabilities (Margalit & Ben-Dov, 1992; Unger, 1992; Zehavi, 1992). These youngsters, who reported experiencing higher levels of loneliness feelings when compared to nondisabled youngsters, were also rated by teachers and mothers as demonstrating more loneliness and lower social skills. In a study of 93 boys with behavior disorders in grades 4 to 8 (Margalit, 1993b), moderately significant negative correlations were found between loneliness and social skills (both self-reported and teacher-rated). These results for behavior disordered children resembled the studies of students with mental retardation and learning disabilities. In order to further investigate the profile of the lonely child with behavior disabilities, the students were divided into two groups: those who reported low loneliness ($n = 47$) and those who reported high levels of loneliness ($n = 46$). The lonely group revealed lower self-reported and teacher-rated social skills and more extreme behavior and learning difficulties.

Social skills deficiencies can be categorized into four basic types, defined according to the child's knowledge of how to perform the behavior in question and the presence or absence of interfering cognitive, emotional or behavioral responses (Elliott, Sheridan, & Gresham, 1989; Gresham, 1981, 1984). The four specific types consist of: skill deficits, performance deficits, self-control skill deficits, and self-control performance deficits. This conceptualization of social skills deficits was influenced by Bandura's (1977) distinction between acquisition and performance deficits. Even when children learn a social response (i.e., acquisition), sufficient experience is needed to ensure the child's ability for age-appropriate application of the mastered skill (i.e., performance). The concept of interfering responses is crucial to the understanding of self-control skills, because it is assumed that responses such as the anger, distraction, and over-excitement typifying disabled children who have difficulties in affective regulation and routinely encounter frustrations, may interfere with the acquisition of social skills and even more with their smooth performance (Elliott, Sheridan, & Gresham, 1989). Children may be able to explain in detail what the desired response should be during peer interactions, and may even have a high level of motivation and promise to behave as expected, with the best and most honest intentions. Yet when facing excitement or frustrations, they may prove unable to perform the socially accepted behavior.

Loneliness and social skills in a reciprocal model

Reciprocal relations exist between social skills and loneliness. An individual lacking in interpersonal skills is less able to initiate, establish, and maintain satisfying relations. But the experience of loneliness may in turn affect the person's sense of competence (Spitzberg & Hurt, 1987). There is some evidence that lonely individuals may be less able to concentrate and to direct their attention effectively toward others (Peplau & Perlman, 1982; Perlman & Peplau, 1982). They are highly self-conscious or self-focused (Jones, Freemon, & Goswick, 1981) and more concerned about themselves than with others and their communicative messages. Weiss (1973) claimed that when lonely individuals do appraise others, it is often only for their potential as providers of the needed relations. In this vein, situations are appraised only for their potential in making the desired relationships available. Thus, loneliness in itself may produce ignorance of crucial social cues, an over-sensitivity to minimal and less significant social cues, and a tendency to misinterpret others' intentions. As loneliness becomes more chronic, social skills become less competent through lack of use and/or through motivational deficits.

Low self-esteem, poor social skills, and high social anxiety may simultaneously be antecedents and outcomes of loneliness. Children who have been rejected by their peer group were found to have deficient social skills when compared with better accepted children (Asher, Parkhurst, Hymel, & Williams, 1990).

Attribution style

The process of providing explanations for loneliness is complex and intimately bound to the individual's construction of social relationships, perception of social situations, and personal motivations (Lunt, 1991). Attribution research has demonstrated that children's social responses are in part determined by their causal interpretations of situations (Dodge, 1983), influencing their affective, motivational, and cognitive responses to life events (Weiner & Handel, 1985). While attributions, or the ways in which individuals explain events, have long been seen to play a central part in determining behavior, they also reflect individual differences in a consistent manner across a variety of situations (Abramson, Seligman, & Teasdale, 1978; Burns & Seligman, 1989; Tiggemann, Winefield, Winefield, & Goldney, 1991). Tiggemann et al. (1991) demonstrated in their studies the stability of attribution style. Those individuals with depressed affect and feelings of hopelessness attributed positive experiences as more externally rooted and as less stable, whereas negative experiences were viewed as more stable and global. Thus, the occurrence and the severity of loneliness feelings may be understood to be related to the kinds of attributions people make regarding their life events (Anderson & Arnoult, 1985; Weiner, 1985).

Another approach (Lunt, 1991) highlighted the need for researchers to map out different self-explanations, suggesting that people do not use a single attribution to explain a situation, but rather utilize a network of attributions that are perceived as related and interlocked together. Lunt's research stressed the importance of focusing on the interconnectedness between the different attributed causes of loneliness and of categorizing these causes according to the position they occupy within the total network. Although the present discussion will elaborate these dimensions separately, it should be remembered that their true significance can be understood only through the study of their networks and connections.

Three major attributional dimensions have been suggested by various researchers (Lunt, 1991; Peplau, Miceli, & Morasch, 1982; Weiner, 1985):

1 *Locus of control.* Attributions can be internal to a person, for example:

"They don't like me because I'm stupid and always give stupid answers"
as compared to those externally or situationally related:
"Those kids don't want me on their team because they've been playing together for more than a year, and I'm new in this neighborhood" or *"He was rude and asked me to leave the room because that day there was an important competition, and he was really tense."*

2 *Stability*. Attributions may be characterized as either changeable, such as:
"Today I better stay home, but tomorrow I'll play with the group"
or stable:
"It always was and always will be like this: Everybody else is out having fun at the party, while I'm at home bored and depressed."

3 *Controllability*. Attributions reflect the person's belief in his or her control over activities and feelings, for example:
"I'll try harder, and eventually they'll appreciate me"
or the lack of control:
"They don't like me, and I can't do anything about it."

Lonely individuals tend to attribute interpersonal failures and successes to uncontrollable, stable factors in their lives more than do non-lonely individuals (Anderson & Arnoult, 1985; Anderson & Riger, 1991). The longer a person experiences loneliness, the more his or her causal explanations will shift from external, unstable, and controllable (situational) causes to internal, stable, and uncontrollable (chronic) causes. The child who attributes loneliness to situational changes (e.g., a new school; separation from good friends) will be more likely to cope with these feelings by seeking new interpersonal contacts. In contrast, chronically lonely children may come to believe that they themselves are the main cause of their loneliness. Children who attribute to themselves personal unattractiveness or a lack of appropriate social skills may gradually persuade themselves of the totality of their difficulties, further reducing the intensity of their coping efforts and their motivation to initiate interactions (Young, 1982).

The network of attributed causes for loneliness should be studied for each of its dimensions and their interrelations. For example, loneliness has been found to be related to a lower desire for intimacy among persons who held generalized external expectations of control (Mikulincer & Segal, 1991). Among those who held internal expectancies of control, loneliness was related to a higher desire for intimacy. Controllability was not found to be a significant predictor of loneliness when combined with other predictor variables such as a self-rated social skills measure (Inderbitzen-Pisaruk, Clark, & Solano, 1992). The gender variable as related to controllability also showed differential relations with loneliness. Males viewed their loneliness as related to their feelings of lower levels of control over their success and failure, but females did not.

The motivational consequences of loneliness can be understood only by taking into account the moderating role of the person's network of control expectancies (Mikulincer & Segal, 1991). When people believe that they have no personal control over the course of environmental events, loneliness has a depressing effect on their desire for relations and intimacy. Lonely people who believe that events are beyond their personal control, appraising themselves as possessing a lower self-efficacy for "making friends," might believe that loneliness cannot be ended by their own actions, and their pessimism might manifest itself in apathy and isolation. In contrast, when people believe that events are subject to their own personal control and are changeable, loneliness has a facilitating effect on the motivation for initiating interrelations. Lonely people who believe that they have personal control over events might believe that they can end their loneliness, reflecting greater hopes and optimism.

Expectancies of control may also be understood as having a moderating role on coping styles and related attributions (Mikulincer & Segal, 1991). On the one hand, problem-centered coping strategies will be adopted by individuals who believe that they have control over events and attribute loneliness to unstable and changeable causes (Solomon, Mikulincer, & Avitzur, 1988). On the other hand, lonely people who believe that they have no control over events might attribute loneliness to stable causes, thus adopting emotion-focused coping strategies, which in turn might produce apathy, depressive mood, and greater isolation.

In summary, the attributed causes of loneliness, especially in terms of their stability, perceived controllability, or personal responsibility (locus of control) seem to guide loneliness-related emotions and behaviors. The mapping out of interrelations among the various beliefs and expectations about others' reactions may clarify personal trends pointing at individual differences. All these traits interact with gender and age variables and may be perceived as related to age- and gender-related social roles and tasks.

Conclusions

This chapter presented research on the personality characteristics of lonely individuals. Research demonstrated that self-perceptions, self-efficacy beliefs, social skills, and attributional styles were consistently related to loneliness, yet were interlocked within an interrelated network of traits that are also linked to gender and age. A simplistic approach may accentuate the fact that children with disabilities, whose personal history of failures in highly valued tasks resulted in lower self-competence, decreased social skills, and a different attributional style to their social difficulties, were found to experience higher levels of loneliness. However, this approach ignores the complexity of the children's network of personality variables.

Loneliness and companionship can be treated as both personal and interpersonal experiences. Individual traits and contextual components alike contribute to human connections and relations. In addition to research on the personal characteristics related to loneliness, the impact of ecological factors has received major research attention. The study of loneliness among students with disabilities requires in-depth investigation directed toward the environmental conditions that promote or limit the child's abilities and the likelihood of experiencing satisfying human relations. The next section will focus on contexts for interpersonal relations, presenting research on two environmental systems in which the child operates: the family and peer contexts.

Section II
Interpersonal Family and Peer Contexts

3 Family Environment

Research has consistently linked aspects of the family environment to features of children's cognitive and emotional functioning that predict social competence (Moos, 1991; Patterson, 1982). In the ordinary course of events, interactions within the family system provide the majority of children with the knowledge and experience that will serve as the basis for social growth and peer relations. At the beginning of life, the infant's development as a separate individual with a coherent identity depends upon interactions between the baby and the parental figure. Early socialization processes in the family gradually shape the child's social behaviors and attitudes. Interpersonal relations, the family climate, parental abilities or difficulties, and other components of family experience have been found to be closely related to children's social functioning. Social development and loneliness have essentially been considered a product of family processes and interactions (Large, 1989; Rubin & Slomon, 1984).

Viewing child-adult interactions as an important determinant in children's development, changes may be expected in the interaction patterns and attachment relations of a family with a disabled infant, with important later consequences on the child's cognitive development and social and emotional skills (Fraser, 1986). These changes in the parent-infant interactions may stem from the baby's special needs due to the disabling condition and/or from the parents' emotional reactions to the realization of having a different child and the additional demands involved in raising a child with special needs. The disability in the family affects the interactions, changing the way the family system operates (Turnbull & Turnbull, 1986).

Yet changes related to a child's disabling condition do not initiate a simply unidirectional modification in the family. Bronfenbrener (1979, 1986) emphasized in his studies the importance of determining the bidirectional influences of persons, settings, and their characteristics on outcome measures. A series of studies based on the transactional-ecological model has demonstrated the bidirectional influence of parent-child relations (Maccoby & Martin, 1983), wherein children's characteristics are seen to influence parental behavior and systemic relations within the family, as much as parents influence their children. Within the transactional model, accepting the family as a system in which each member affects and is affected by others, this chapter will attempt to provide a review of current trends in research on families with disabled children, with a focus on areas that promote the children's social interrelations and on how the child's loneliness relates to these specific family aspects.

Different approaches to loneliness such as social learning, psychodynamic, and developmental orientations were involved in a search focused on the family environment to find what can go wrong in the process of personality development, in order to understand those individuals who suffer from a failure in establishing and maintaining satisfactory and meaningful interpersonal relationships. Social learning theory takes the position that social behavior is learned in the family as a social setting. Youngsters are viewed as acquiring at least some of their social behavioral repertoire through their interactions with their parents (Coie, 1990). The social skills learned in their early interactions with parents are later generalized to different interaction styles with peers (East, 1991). Learning can occur through various processes such as modeling, reinforcement, and direct instruction of behavioral rules within and outside the family system (Jolligg & Horne, 1986). The social learning approach (Asher, 1983; Ladd, 1988) has focused much interest on current group interactions and friendships, and on peer acceptance and rejection as predictors of loneliness experiences. Children's disabilities, so often manifested by learning difficulties, may prevent the normal acquisition of social skills through learning.

The psychodynamic orientation focuses interest on the needs of young children and the quality of interrelations between them and their parents. The infant's early development was studied as a predictor of loneliness experiences in adult life (Bowlby, 1973; Winnicott, 1965). During infancy, the child's emotional demands for affection, companionship, and stimulating intimacy must be answered by the parent in a reliable and regular pattern (Goldstein, Freud, & Solnit, 1979). Solnit (1986) emphasized the importance of the parent as the auxiliary ego of the child, until the child's ego capacities develop sufficiently to take over the needed mediating, regulating functions of environmental information. According to Mahler's conceptualizations (Mahler, Pine, & Bergman, 1975), the infant is viewed as part of a symbiotic tie with the mother and is psychologically merged with her. Development thus becomes a process of separation, of creating boundaries, and of developing an independent self. On the other hand, Stern's (1985) view of the baby as a separate and helpless individual implied a developmental process where constant attempts are necessary to learn varied ways for interacting with different persons in the environment.

Researchers of human development within the psychodynamic orientation have thus focused their studies on different aspects of children's connections, separation, and loneliness within the family, highlighting two opposing trends in human interrelatedness -- toward developing closeness to other people and toward developing a distance by becoming self-sufficient and independent of others (Storr, 1988). Each child is considered an individual who, from birth, is separate from others yet constantly attempts to develop meaningful relations. There are many ways for children to make connections, to reach through the space that separates people (Josselson, 1992). Close and intimate ties must be established with some people, whereas more superficial relations must be developed with others. As children grow, they learn to better differentiate the complex and varied ways of relating to and maintaining separateness from others. Within this approach, the slow developmental pace and special needs of children with disabilities can be expected to affect the children's establishment of intimate relations and their separation process, reducing parents' confidence as to when to enhance and when to delay their children's attempts at independence.

The developmental approach emphasizes the transactions between the youngsters and their families at different age stages. For example, adolescents' expectations for greater autonomy and responsibility are closely related to parental ability to give more freedom and autonomy and to the youngsters' greater involvement with their peer group (Petersen, 1988). Parents of disabled children treat their children as younger than their chronological age, reflecting overprotection and anxiety (Margalit, 1984). Parents often feel that expectations for independence and autonomy for their children lead to early exposure to social tasks and responsibilities for which they might not be ready.

These different approaches all explore the role of the family in children's successful social development or their failure to establish satisfactory social relations. The critical interrelations within the family system do not constitute a stable, unchanging entity, but rather reflect distinct patterns at different developmental stages (Weiss, 1987). Various types of relationships meet the different interpersonal needs or offer the distinct "social provisions" (Weiss, 1974) that the child requires throughout the course of development. Changing needs and different social tasks characterize each developmental stage (Sullivan, 1953). When disabilities affect children's developmental paths, these needs may be expressed differently.

Stages in connectedness

Josselson's (1992) model integrated the psychodynamic and developmental perspectives, identifying eight primary relation patterns during development in which people overcome the distance between them in order to develop satisfying relations. Each pattern involves, actually or metaphorically, a way of reaching or being reached that emerges from the individual's developmental stage, ranging from concrete and basic experiences to more symbolic and complex ones. This model is considered valuable for understanding the process of normal and atypical development.

Holding

Holding is the first interpersonal experience for the baby, representing security and basic trust (Josselson, 1992). Within infant-adult interrelations, a *powerful arm* keeps the child from falling, protecting the child from an anxiety-provoking and fearful experience. Winnicott's (1965) conceptualization of the origin of loneliness emphasized the important role of the *holding mother* who provides a safe environment for the baby in which to experiment within her presence. Winnicott suggested that the achievement of a capacity to stay alone may be an important stage in development that originates with the infant's experience of being alone in the presence of the mother.

For children with disabilities, the sources of the loneliness experience may originate in their inability to stay alone. During normal growth, infants need to develop a recognition of the dependable existence of adult support, if their sense of being a separate individual with a separate identity is to develop. Winnicott assumed that this begins to happen when the infant experiences the sense of being alone, while remaining in a relaxed state and feeling assured of the presence and availability of the mother. Although, as Storr (1988) stated, Winnicott's suppositions about the subjective experiences of infants are impossible to prove, Storr found them important for illuminating the developmental task of staying alone. Winnicott suggested that the capacity to be alone is also related to children's ability to get in touch with themselves, to discover what they need or want irrespective of what others expect from them, and to express their inner feelings. Children with disabilities, as a result of their limited capacities, may not be able to attend to the supportive, confident adult or to benefit from this relationship.

The capacity to be alone may be conceptualized as a sign of inner security, rather than as an expression of a withdrawn state. Winnicott assumed that in order to move away from the mother, to develop separateness, and to actively explore the environment, the baby must have already internalized a sense of being "held" adequately, of feeling secure.

The concepts of supportive relationships and social supports have emerged as a major focus of research on stress and resources. The attempt to clarify social support processes can be compared to a study of the mature experience of symbolic holding (Vaux, 1987). Children who feel safe and protected within the family's boundaries are able to internalize what Erickson (1968) called a sense of basic trust that enables them to experiment and learn within their later environments.

Attachment

Similar to Weiss' (1973, 1974) social provisions construct, attachment has been suggested as the second type of relatedness (Josselson, 1992). Attachment focuses attention on a different set of relations than holding. We can develop attachment to people who have not held us, and we can be held by people to whom we are not attached. While the opposite of holding is falling, the opposite of attachment is aloneness. The two concepts are interrelated but not identical. Attachment refers to the experience of togetherness and emotional linkage -- the assurance that, if needed, intimacy and closeness will be available. Being held is a passive situation, whereas attachment is an active process of getting closer to someone, actually or symbolically, to reduce anxiety (Josselson, 1992).

This model highlighted the need to enhance awareness of the togetherness concept in order to develop in the child the roots for later interpersonal intimacy. The quality of infant-parent attachment and interactions has been consistently associated with the later development of satisfactory interactions with peers (Cassidy, Parke, Butkovsky, & Braungart, 1992; LaFreniere & Sroufe, 1985). Attachment theorists relate overt behaviors to internal processes, through the assessment of infants' behavior when observed separating from mothers in different situational conditions (Ainsworth, 1990). Attachment has been defined as an interactive process in which mother and infant each affect one another, thus reflecting the quality of the emotional ties within the mother-child unit (Fraser, 1986; Winnicott, 1965). Bowlby (1988) characterized early emotional bonds as attachments that serve a critical function in providing a secure base for children throughout their growth. Attachment has been often considered to be a vital process in human ontogeny, viewing it not only as a developmental task that must be successfully resolved, but also as a continual expression of the adaptation process (Cicchetti, Cummings, Greenberg, & Marvin, 1990).

Research on emotional isolation as one dimension of loneliness has been influenced by Bowlby's (1973, 1988) concepts of attachment. Bowlby differentiated between attachment and dependence. Dependence is at its maximum at birth, when the infant is most helpless and in need of support or a holding arm (Josselson, 1992). Gradually, this dependence diminishes until maturity is reached. If an adult is considered dependent, this implies immaturity. In contrast, attachment behavior persists throughout the life of a well-adjusted person. If a person does not have intimate attachments, this is usually considered a sign of emotional difficulties. Children with disabilities may be considered helpless, dependent, and vulnerable, and their parents, through their dedication and concern, may attempt to provide protection, support, and even overprotection of their children, thus further influencing the children's independence and ability to form attachments.

Additional relation patterns

Weiss' (1974) discussion of relationship provisions explored the individual's need for reassurance of worth, provided by relationships in which the person's skills and abilities are acknowledged. Josselson (1992) viewed the roots of this relation in the mother-infant eye-to-eye mode of relations. In eye-to-eye relating is the recognition that we have meaning to others. This need to matter to others has a psychological significance as an aspect of forming a sense of self in relation to the world. The eye-to-eye mode is closely related to peer acceptance and/or rejection. This aspect may be a source of difficulty for children with disabilities, whose deficient functioning can be translated into lower self-efficacy as well as parents' stressful reactions.

Idealization and identification as modes of connectedness are ways of linking ourselves to powerful members of the community, striving to become like them or to control them. Weiss (1974) refers to this provision as a search for guidance, leading to relationships with trustworthy and authoritative individuals who can provide advice and assistance.

In contrast with attachment relations, passionate relations have been less emphasized by theoreticians, but their value cannot be minimized. Josselson (1992) proposed that passionate experience within the relationship construct is related to the child's emotional arousal and claim for attention and love. Passion is expressed more through its intensity, whereas the nature of the connection (intimate close friendship, love) may be less important.

A more mature means of connectedness is companionship involving a sense of mutuality, such as when a child stands side by side with someone, creating a bond that is the product of both children, an emergent "group" concept (Josselson, 1992). Weiss (1973) put forth the similar concept of reliable alliance, derived from relationships in which the person can count on assistance. Mutuality exists on a continuum of sharing experiences, ranging from simple alliances to deeply intimate relationships. In describing companionship relationships, people tend to focus not on the nature of the activity in which the parties are involved, but rather on the togetherness experience itself (Josselson, 1992). Related to the companionship formation is the important emergence of a "we" feeling or experience, a sense of being one part that fits into a larger entity. Similar to Weiss' (1974) "social integration" concept, provided by the network of relationships in which individuals share interests and concerns, Josselson (1992) extended her discussion to the experience of belonging to a group. This dimension of embeddedness in a group enables one to feel included and differentiated at the same time, to experience communality and belonging, individuality and independence. Children who wish to belong but do not belong to the peer group, have an intense feeling of being left out, of social isolation. Children with disabilities want to be a part of the peer group but are often rejected. Research on acceptance and rejection within the peer group may add important clarification to the loneliness construct.

A fully mature type of relations is expressed through nurturance relations. The developing child, even the one with difficulties and disabilities, must learn to take care of others. Weiss (1974) also recognized this relational need for providing nurturance, derived from relationships in which the person feels responsible for the well-being of another who needs help and support. This type of relationship has special value for the child who demonstrates excessive caring needs and constantly expects support and help. Without careful intervention planning, such a child may not develop an ability to see and care for others' needs, in order to support his or her own personal values, importance, and resourcefulness.

For methodological purposes, the different modes of relationships presented above were described separately. However, it is well accepted that in any type of relationship, several dimensions may be involved simultaneously or sequentially. Interrelations may be conceptualized as independent and/or as inter-penetrating and incorporating each other. The emphasis on self (autonomy, self-control, independence) seems to contradict the basic need for others (relatedness, affection, and responsiveness). Yet, Josselson's (1992) multidimensional construct did not view relatedness and individuality as dichotomous. Developmental processes concern both maintaining ties with others and at the same time maintaining differentiation from others.

Recent research has been directed toward a reconceptualization of the attachment construct, attempting to clarify the role of the interrelations between parents (especially mothers) and their children who have unique abilities and disabilities in the development of later loneliness and social competence (Ainsworth, 1990).

Early relations and disabilities

From the early stages of development, the need for human intimacy appears and finds its expression in the infant's desire for continuous contact with the parents. Recent research pointed out that attachment is an extended and dynamic process continuing throughout the life cycle. Children are continually renegotiating the balance between being connected to others and being independent and autonomous as they encounter new developmental phases. Once an attachment develops, it continues to undergo transformations and reintegrations with subsequent accomplishments such as emerging autonomy and entrance into the peer world (Cicchetti, Cummings, Greenberg, & Marvin, 1990; Cummings, 1990).

A mother approaches her newborn baby with certain assumptions and beliefs about the infant's needs and abilities and her competencies and priorities as a mother. Her assumptions and expectations are reinforced by signals from the baby, indicating to the mother her importance to the baby. If the mother's perceptions of the infant's needs and abilities are limited, due to her emotional stress or her perception of the child's disability and/or slow development, the child may receive a restricted input, too little attention, and a limited range of shared parent-child activities (Fraser, 1986). These interactions with the parent can be assumed to further impede the disabled child's social growth and to contribute to the child's later development of loneliness feelings. Neglect, like unwilling separation or loss during childhood, may develop into relational problems in later years. On the other hand, too much emotional closeness -- fusion or intrusion -- may result in a similar deficit in the ability to form the kind of socio-emotional bond that prevents emotional isolation.

The concept of intrusion in the socialization experience seems to be related to a combination of family isolation and excessive emotional warmth within the family, leading to parental overprotection. This concept has special importance for children with disabilities, who often experience parental love that is overcontrolling and overprotecting, as a reflection of parental anxiety, thus further inhibiting the child's exploratory activities in the environment. The result of this mode of socialization is that the child experiences difficulties in becoming differentiated from one or both parents and in developing a self-identity as an autonomous person. When a young child has an exaggerated sense of self, life consists of complete love, attention, and admiration. Emotional bonding with others then becomes impossible, and there is a growing risk of loneliness (Andersson, 1990).

The recognition of the bidirectional nature of the influence between the nonsatisfying parent-child bonding relationship and the child's interpersonal difficulties, whether manifested by withdrawal or aggression, underscores the need to use a transactional perspective (East, 1991).

In summary, when the normal path of development is hampered through the child's disabilities, different attachment patterns may be developed. The infant-parent interrelations not only reflect an attempt to meet the greater and more critical needs of the child, but also the parents' lower ability to mediate the increased environmental demands due to their own emotional distressful reactions to the birth and care of their handicapped child, often leading to greater parental overprotection and intrusion.

Children's disabilities and parental stress

The pioneering research by Farber in the late 1950's revealed that family members experience significant stress in raising their children with severe mental retardation (Farber, 1959). Researchers, theoreticians, and clinicians in the past decades have begun to conceive of children's developmental outcomes as having multiple causal determinants rather than as single-factor etiologies (Cummings & Cicchetti, 1990). The outgrowth of this thinking is conceptualized in the transactional model, viewing the multiple connections among environmental forces, parental characteristics, and child characteristics as dynamic reciprocal contributions to the course of the child's development (Cummings & Cicchetti, 1990). Parental appraisal of stress and handicapping conditions, the availability of resources such as support networks, and the power and flexibility to adapt coping strategies and respond appropriately to children's needs are important mediators of the children's social-emotional development in families with disabled children (McCubbin & Patterson, 1983). The stress-resources-coping paradigm has commonly been presented as a working model for understanding parents with disabled children.

Stress-resources-coping model

Within the stress-resources-coping paradigm, different researchers have concentrated their efforts on identifying a variety of factors that might increase or decrease parental stress and on defining meaningful interrelations to explain their coping. This model recalls that families with children who have disabilities are not basically different from other families, yet they can be expected to face increased amounts of stress, to experience greater demands on their personal and familial resources, and to respond with more avoidance and less active coping mechanisms. Childhood disability makes increased demands on families' resources in terms of individual and systemic resources (Seligman & Darling, 1989).

The experience of stress emerges when the demands made on fathers and mothers with a disabled child, originating in their internal and/or external environments, exceed their personal and family resources and are not met by available, automatic, and adaptive responses (Antonovsky, 1979, 1987). Research surveys pointed out that parents of children with disabilities often report experiencing more stress than do parents of children without disabilities (Boyce, Behl, Mortensen, & Akers, 1991; Burden & Thomas, 1986; Friedrich & Friedrich, 1981; Kazak & Marvin, 1984; Wilton & Renault, 1986). The picture emerging from parental reports among families of disabled children, using different samples and research instruments, is one of extreme fatigue due to increased demands for time investment and constant attempts to meet the many demands on financial, physical, and emotional resources, regarding not only parents but also every member of the family. An understanding of the predominant experience of stress in families with disabled children and of their resources to cope with the exceptional demands they face is essential to the conceptualization of the family system's impact on the child's social growth and loneliness.

Sources of stress

The sources of parental stress following the diagnosis of disabilities in their children may be a combined product of the increased caring needs of the child and the emotional reactions of the parents. Parents' emotional reactions have been categorized into a three-factor model (Eden-Piercy, Blacher, & Eyman, 1986):

1. Shock-guilt-despair reactions, with expressions such as *"I feel that having a handicapped child like this is the biggest tragedy of my life."*

2. Refusal-denial reactions, with statements such as *"I'm sure my child will catch up, she doesn't seem handicapped."*

3. Recovery-acceptance reactions, with expressions such as *"I feel I am not to blame for my child's problems"* or *"Some people stare at my child, but that's only because they're curious."*

Stressful feelings in parents of disabled children were found to be interrelated both with the parents' individual characteristics and with the family's systemic resources (Folkman, Schaefer, & Lazarus, 1979; Friedrich, Wilturner, & Cohen, 1985). Some aspects of parental stress were found to be more specifically associated with children's characteristics (e.g., clinical category, severity of handicapping condition, presence of additional behavior and health problems) and with the availability of family resources such as community support systems. Other aspects of parental stress have been highlighted consistently for different handicapping conditions within different cultures such as in the USA, Japan, Israel, and Germany (Dumas, 1986; Dyson & Fewell, 1986; Friedrich, Wilturner, & Cohen, 1985; Hofmann, 1983; Margalit, Leyser, Ankonina, & Avraham, 1991; Margalit, Leyser, Avraham, & Lewy-Osin, 1988; Mullins, 1987; Nimi & Uemura, 1987).

Research has indicated that mothers may be more affected by the additional stressors related to caring for a disabled child than are the other family members. Several studies have reported that mothers of disabled children experience significantly more feelings of personal distress, bear responsibility for most of the caring functions in the family, experience fewer and less rewarding social interactions, and have significantly less free time (Breiner & Young, 1985; Bristol, Gallagher, & Schopler, 1988; Hofmann, 1983; Kazak, 1987). The fact that professionals often expect these mothers to take on many new roles related to the child's disabilities (such as being their children's tutors, trainers, and therapists) may result in increasing their therapeutic abilities for short-term interventions, yet can diminish the ability to function in the long-run as accepting and supporting mothers whose interrelations with their infants may provide the basis for later social-emotional growth.

An example of one source of stress due to the disabling condition that was often reported by parents and is closely related to the loneliness research consists of the children's free time and leisure activities. Parents often discuss their children's difficulties in planning and spending their free time in an enjoyable and age-appropriate manner. Even during school years, when most children are almost independent in their free-time activities, parents of children with disabilities reported that they must continue to plan and supervise their children's leisure activities. This results not only in parental feelings of overload and fatigue, but also in a pronounced impact on the children's social growth and independence.

A survey of leisure activities among learning disabled students (Margalit, 1984) revealed their tendency to be involved in passive, adult-dependent activities that were often evaluated as suitable for younger children. According to distressed parents' reports, disabled children often complain that when they are not participating in school or structured activities, they feel bored and await adult proposals of free-time activities. In contrast to most nondisabled children, who gradually develop independent activities, many students with disabilities require a prolonged period of adult supervision, instruction, and guidance in order to foster the development of meaningful and satisfying leisure activities. This extended dependence reflects not only the children's increased need for adult guidance, but also the delay in their development of an ability to stay alone (Winnicott, 1965).

In understanding the many pathways to the development and perpetuation of feelings of loneliness within children who have disabilities, the transactional model may be useful by presenting a network of factors that intertwine from the early developmental stages. Among the participants in transactional processes, three major factors can be identified: those characteristics related to the child, those reflecting parental resources, and those typifying the family's functioning. The children's attributes encompass those related to their disabling conditions and to personality features.

Child characteristics

In line with the conceptualization of the child's disability as a major source of parental crisis, the type and severity level of the handicapping condition were clearly expected to differentiate the amount of stress reported by families. Higher levels of parental stress have been found in families with a disabled child as related to the severity of the child's difficulties (Breen & Barkley, 1988; Friedrich, Wilturner, & Cohen, 1985) and, more specifically, to the child's slower rate of progress, more difficult temperament, and lower social responsiveness (Gallagher, Beckman, & Cross, 1985). Different levels of maternal concern were found when mothers of children with Down's syndrome were compared to mothers of children with motor impairments, calling for the utilization of a more handicap-specific pattern of maternal emotional reactions, in order to foster individualized intervention planning (Hodapp, Dykens, Evans, & Merighi, 1992).

Friedrich, Wilturner, and Cohen (1985) also found a relation between the child's behavior problems and the level of family stress. This relation has been considered bidirectional, with parents' distress contributing to the behavioral problems of their handicapped children and vice versa. Evidence has been presented for a reciprocal effect between ineffective parenting, especially in the area of discipline, and the child's disruptive behavior, pinpointing that they mutually maintain one another (Vuchinich, Bank, & Patterson, 1992). A relationship between children's temperament and mothers' adjustment was also found, with mothers of temperamentally difficult preschool children reporting more psychosocial difficulties. The mothers were more prone to anxiety, depressive mood, and doubts about their competence as parents. These mothers reported that they felt less emotionally close to their children, and found that their parenting role restricted their lives to a greater extent (Sheeber & Johnson, 1992).

Feelings of anxiety were more common among mothers of children with childhood psychosis than in mothers of children with motor-handicaps or Down's syndrome (Ryde-Brandt, 1990). Boyce, Behl, Mortensen, and Akers' (1991) study with a large sample of 479 families demonstrated that the functioning level of the children (including their ability to take care of themselves, relate and communicate with others, and perform motor and cognitive functions) had the strongest effect on child-related stress but not on maternally-related stress. Yet the severity of the child's handicapping condition provides only a partial explanation for the family's functioning style and coping abilities (Blacher, Nihira, & Meyers, 1987).

Studies of mother-child interactions comparing normal children and different groups of children with disabilities such as hyperactivity, language-delays, and general delays, identified major stressors in families of disabled children as related specifically to the impact of the severity of the children's handicaps on parent-child interactions (Siegel & Cunningham, 1984). Parents responded differently to the developmentally delayed and disabled infants. When the developmentally delayed infant failed to provide the appropriate cues for parental behavior, the parent responded with stimulation considered inadequate for development. The developmentally delayed child thus becomes even more delayed due to the non-optimal environment, and gradually it becomes even harder for the parent to provide the appropriate stimulation in the family environment (Siegel & Cunningham, 1984). The language-delayed children, for example, initiated fewer of the conversational teaching exchanges that may contribute to cognitive and social-emotional development. The overactive, inattentive, noncompliant behavior of the attention deficit disordered children prompted their parents to use more controlling behavior, which may perpetuate these children's behavior difficulties. The developmentally delayed children initiated fewer interactions, were less responsive to adults, and prompted a pattern of increased parental dominance that may compound the children's lack of social initiative. Thus, the consequence of different child characteristics due to the type and severity of the handicapping condition can be expected to be the development of different patterns of mother-child attachment. The behavioral control, socialization processes, and emotional regulation of the mother-child dyad may be impaired, further affecting parental feelings of competence and thus parents' ability to foster their children's social growth.

Parental characteristics

Within the transactional model, personality dispositions of fathers and mothers, in terms of self-efficacy, self-confidence, and perceived control were all found to be related to effective coping with the child's handicapping condition. Perceived self-efficacy reflects parental beliefs in their capacity to increase the motivation, cognitive assets, and path of action necessary to help their children with and without disabilities. These judgements of personal efficacy affect their choices of activities and regulate their efforts (Bandura & Wood, 1989; Ozer & Bandura, 1990). Parents who expect that a given behavior will lead to the desired outcome -- enhancing the growth of their children with disabilities -- and that they are capable of performing these actions, will feel and behave differently than parents who feel ineffective and helpless where their children's development is concerned. Mothers who considered themselves to be capable, and to possess the capacity to make changes, reported better functioning (Friedrich, Wilturner, & Cohen, 1985).

Parental belief systems and values regarding social relations on the one hand, and their attitudes toward the disability and expectations from the child with disabilities on the other hand, may affect their interactions and reactions to the child's difficulties, and especially to the child's social failures and feelings of loneliness. Parent-child interactions during different play activities, parental beliefs, and parents' disciplinary style have all been found to be related to their children's peer competence (Gottman & Fainsilber Katz, 1989; Hart, Ladd, & Burleson, 1990; Pettit, Dodge, & Brown, 1988). Four groups of personality characteristics have been conceptualized as having powerful links with the mediation of stressors such as those encountered by parents of disabled children:

1. Personal coherence
2. Emotional functioning
3. Coping style
4. Access to social support

Parental sense of coherence

A global personality construct such as the sense of coherence (Antonovsky, 1987; Antonovsky & Sourani, 1988) provides an important index of parental functioning, within a salutogenic model focusing on the healthy rather than pathological facets of personality. Parental sense of coherence can be defined as a global orientation that expresses the extent to which parents have confidence that their internal and external environments can be viewed and treated as structured and predictable; that resources are available to meet the increased demands; and that these demands can be considered challenges worthy of energy investment and engagement. Sense of coherence was conceptualized as consisting of three interrelated components:

1 Comprehensibility
2 Manageability
3 Meaningfulness

Comprehensibility refers to the extent to which one perceives environmental information as ordered, consistent, and structured, rather than as unpredictable, disordered, and accidental. Parents with a high sense of comprehensibility expect to be able to predict what will happen in the future, and even expect surprises to be explicable when they appear.

Manageability defines the extent to which parents expect that their available resources will meet demands. These resources may lie under the parent's own control or may be available from others as the need develops, such as the support and help of professionals or friends.

Meaningfulness represents the affective-motivational aspect of personal coherence. Parents who view many events and activities as challenging and as worthy of emotional investment and commitment are considered as having a strong meaningfulness level.

Consistent research findings have pointed out that parents with a disabled child reported lower measures of coherence (Margalit, Leyser, Avraham, & Lewy-Osin, 1988; Margalit, Raviv, & Ankonina, 1992) when compared to parents without disabled children. Although coherence may be viewed as a relatively stable personality trait, parenting a child with disabilities was found to have a pronounced impact on parents' confidence that future life events will be predictable and sensible and will work out as well as can be expected. Parental inability to identify a meaningful answer to the critical question "Why is this happening to us?" often leads to a decreased feeling of control and confidence in the environment, resulting in a lower sense of coherence. Emotional functioning is a construct closely related to coherence, with significance for understanding those characteristics of parents with disabled children that may have an important impact on the family environment.

Parental affect

Children with disabilities may need greater parental support and help to foster their social-emotional growth. Parents who have higher levels of energy and persistence can better model and teach interpersonal relations to their children. Yet parents with disabled children reported increased levels of negative affect (Margalit & Ankonina, 1991) and depressed mood (Friedrich, Wilturner, & Cohen, 1985).

Within the two-factor construct of positive and negative affect, it should be noted that although parents with a disabled child expressed more negative affect than did parents with non-handicapped children, no significant differences were found between parents of children with and without disabilities with regard to their positive affect (Clark & Watson, 1988; Forgas, Bower, & Krantz, 1984; Margalit & Ankonina, 1991). Positive affect, reflecting the extent to which a person feels an active and enthusiastic involvement in some areas of life, is considered important for understanding mental health and well-being (Clark & Watson, 1988; Diener & Emmons, 1984; Forgas & Bower, 1987), highlighting the need to incorporate the affective dimension into intervention planning.

Assuming that families provide the first environment where children learn about emotional rules (i.e., when and how to express your feelings in acceptable and unacceptable manners) and that the regulation of emotions is an important factor in peer relations (Denham, 1986), the evaluation of the emotional expressiveness between parents and children has been used as a measure of family functioning (Cassidy, Parke, Butkovsky, & Braungart, 1992). Mothers' affective reactions can be regarded as a means of emotional socialization, modeling feelings through providing patterns and timing of emotional expressions. Maternal emotions may fulfill emotion-specific communicative functions by showing the children the emotional valence and intensity of certain experiences, by modeling the specific emotions appropriate to an occasion, and by serving as potentially important interpersonal regulators of children's social-emotional development (Cummings, Zahn-Waxler, & Radke-Yarrow, 1981; Denham, 1989; Denham, Zahn-Waxler, Cummings, & Iannotti, 1991).

Denham's (1989) research underscored the relations between maternal affect, especially displays of anger and sadness, and children's social-emotional development and competence. It should be remembered that these relations are bidirectional in the mother-child system (Denham, 1989; Patterson, 1980). Among parents who were found to be warm and responsive to their children's needs, the children were generally more competent with peers and friends. Temperamental traits generally corresponding to expressed emotions in infants showed a relative stability across times and situations (Rothbart, 1986). Temperamentally "difficult" children may elicit more angry reactions from mothers, whereas "easy" infants may enable mothers to exhibit more smiles and more happy and satisfied reactions (Denham, 1989).

According to the transactional model, both children's and mothers' temperamental traits influence the emotions they show in dyadic interactions. Parents who express more distressed emotions and infants who evidence a more difficult temperament may transactionally increase each other's distressed mood. Each of the dyad member's emotions influence the other's emotional responses during interactions, and in time, feed into the child's psychosocial functioning and social-emotional competence. Both the children's temperament and the expressiveness of the family climate jointly contribute to the future social functioning of the child. The coping style of these parents further clarifies their modes of functioning.

Parental coping

Coping can be defined as the thoughts and behaviors used by an individual in evaluating the cognitive and emotional meanings of stressors such as raising a disabled child, and in initiating activities to decrease their impact (Billings & Moos, 1981; Folkman & Lazarus, 1988; Lazarus & Folkman, 1984). Although coping style has been shown to be related to contextual factors and to individual characteristics, it is well accepted that more coping strategies of different types are commonly initiated upon confrontation with stressful environments (Folkman & Lazarus, 1985; Holahan & Moos, 1987a, 1987b; Litt, 1988; Moos, Cronkite, Billings, & Finney, 1987).

Two major groups of coping behaviors have been identified, and each group has been investigated in terms of its impact on aspects of personal adjustment:

1 Active coping strategies, including different methods to actively confront the sources of stress (e.g., information seeking, problem solving).

2 Avoidant coping strategies, constituting efforts to deny, minimize, or escape the stressful situation.

Carver, Scheier and Weintraub (1989) found that, although the two types of coping strategies are mutually related, individuals who perceived their situation as amendable to change reported engaging in more active coping. Subjects whose situation was appraised as uncontrollable and unchangeable reported higher levels of denial and disengagement from activity. Active coping has been related in research to adaptation and well-being, whereas avoidant coping has been related to psychological distress and dissatisfaction (Holahan & Moos, 1985; Kobasa, 1982; Margalit, 1990a).

Margalit and Ankonina (1991) compared 71 couples (fathers and mothers) with a disabled child to 77 couples with nondisabled children, demonstrating that parents of disabled children reported a greater use of avoidance as a coping style and felt less coherent and more distressed. The positive affect of the parents with disabled children was related to parental active coping and to a family climate seen as supportive of interrelations within this system and as encouraging of increased opportunities for the personal growth of its members. An increased use of avoidance coping in families with and without disabled children predicted higher levels of negative and distressed parental affect, pinpointing the crucial maladaptive role played by parents' attempts to deny a stressful reality.

Parental active coping is often expressed through requesting and allocating help and support outside the family. Research focusing on the availability of social and community support has emphasized its importance for the growth and well-being of the family members.

Parental access to social support

Extrafamilial social support is considered a major resource for meeting individual and family needs (Dunst, Trivette, & Deal, 1988; Friedrich, Wilturner, & Cohen, 1985). Social support has even been defined as the information leading individuals to believe that they are cared for, esteemed, and members of a network with mutual obligations. The study of the development of children's loneliness highlighted the need to clarify sources of the parents' own feelings of isolation and alienation and to explore parental attitudes toward social interrelations and support (Lobdell & Perman, 1986).

Four types of social support have been identified (Cohen & Wills, 1985; Dunst, Trivette, & Deal, 1988):

Companionship
Emotional support
Information
Material help

Companionship and emotional support refer to spending time with others together, feeling mutually close, expressing appreciation, and regarding the person as valued. Material support is related to the provision of resources and actual assistance, whereas informational support involves advice and counseling. The support and assistance may be provided in different styles such as formal help (e.g., psychologists, teachers) and informal support (e.g., a friend, another parent).

Most social support research has investigated the type and style of the different supports, with a recent emphasis on the importance of the characteristics of the parent who is receiving the help. In order to take advantage of available possibilities within the community, the parent must be able to accept help and to maintain interpersonal relations. The study of satisfaction from the support provides an important index regarding not only the quality of the support provided, but also the ability of the parent to cope effectively with his or her own loneliness and to benefit from that support (Dunst, Trivette, & Deal, 1988). Only a few studies have investigated parental isolation, but the results were consistent. Negative correlations were found between the availability of social support and mothers' feelings of loneliness (Florian & Krulik, 1991).

In addition to parental characteristics such as personal coherence, affective responses, coping style, and access to social support, that have been attributed with a significant role in conceptualizing family environments, the continued search for stress-resistance factors among families of disabled children has led researchers to examine resources within the family ecology (Crnic, Friedrich, & Greenberg, 1983; Wallander, Varni, Babani, Banis, & Wilcox, 1988).

Family characteristics

Recent research has not only channeled interest toward the parents' sources of stress and characteristics, but has also highlighted the family's strengths and capacity for successful adjustment even under these stressful conditions (Darling, 1988; Rodger, 1987; Trivette, Dunst, Deal, Hamer, & Propst, 1990; Widerstrom & Dudley-Marling, 1986). The latter paradigm concentrates its investigation on those factors which may either exacerbate feelings of stress or may serve a stress-resistance role that empowers family coping (Avison & Turner, 1988; Crnic, Greenberg, Ragozin, Robinson, & Basham, 1983; Friedrich, Wilturner, & Cohen, 1985; Holahan & Moos, 1985; Margalit, 1990a). With a focus on the child characteristics and parental variables as they interact in a transactional way, affecting one another, two major groups of factors may be identified: those contributing to increased feelings of stress and those serving as buffering mechanisms which mediate the effects of stressful life events (Crnic, Friedrich, & Greenberg, 1983; McCubbin & Patterson, 1983).

Two major approaches to family characteristics have been applied to families of disabled children:

1. The family climate model
2. The family functioning or strengths model

Domains within family climate

The family atmosphere or climate has been widely held to mediate the adjustment of its members (Folkman, Schaefer, & Lazarus, 1979). The fact that different aspects of family functioning are closely related to peer status and friendship relations focuses attention onto the climate of families with disabled children and interactional aspects.

The social-ecological model of family climate proposed by Moos and Moos (1976, 1983, 1986) assesses family environment in terms of three underlying domains:

1. Relationship
2. Personal growth
3. System maintenance

The relationship domain refers to the manner in which family members develop meaningful relations where they are involved with and supportive of one another. This domain consists of assessments of the extent to which the family members are close to each other, supportive, and feel commitment to one another. The relationship domain also deals with expressions of positive affect and conflicts.

The personal growth domain assesses the underlying goals toward which the family system is oriented and the extent to which opportunities are available for its individual members to pursue personal goals and interests. This domain refers to the extent to which the family members feel independent, self-sufficient, and assertive. It expresses a competitive and achievement-oriented framework and the degree of interest in social, intellectual, and recreational activities.

The system maintenance domain reflects the degree of structure, organization, and control within the family system. It reflects the degree of openness to change or rigidity tendencies, as well as the family rules and habits.

Research on family ecology (Moos, 1987, 1991) found that more supportive relationships and a greater emphasis on personal growth are linked with family members' increased adjustment and fewer complaints of physical or emotional symptoms. In contrast, rigidity and restrictiveness with regard to the family's system maintenance were found to be correlated with family members' maladjustment.

Some specific associations between aspects of family environment and children's personality and behavior have also been identified by research. Moos (1991) found that adolescents in more cohesive, expressive, and well-organized families were found to be more likely to report a higher sense of well-being and self-esteem and to exhibit greater sociability. Olson (1986), within the three central dimensions of his Circumplex model of families -- Cohesion, Communication, and Adaptability -- also pinpointed higher cohesion in family climate as related to youngsters' better functioning. In a closer, more involved family, children's needs were viewed as more likely to be addressed. Nelson (1984) also demonstrated that cohesive, well-organized families tended to promote their children's adjustment. Similarly, Putallaz and Hope Heflin (1990) described the ways in which parents can influence their children's social development by establishing a cohesive and supportive family environment. In contrast, youth with an extraversive maladaptive (e.g., aggressive) behavior style were shown to be much more likely to belong to families who demonstrated a high level of conflict and who lacked cohesion, expressiveness, and a social orientation (Haddad, Barocas, & Hollenbeck, 1991; McGee, Williams, & Silva, 1984; Patterson & Reid, 1984).

Family climate and disabilities

Studies on families with disabled children reported less supportive, less connected, and more distant family interrelations and a decrease in social and recreational activities, within a more rigid and restrictive household (Margalit & Heiman, 1984, 1986; Margalit, Leyser, Ankonina, & Avraham, 1991; Margalit & Raviv, 1983; Prage, Greenbaum, Silver, Friedman, Kutash, & Duchnowski, 1992). Family relations revealed restricted levels of emotional expression and limited opportunities for conflict resolution. Fewer opportunities were available in the family to pursue personal activities or to enhance the personal growth of its members.

Another aspect of the lower family cohesion was expressed by the greater discrepancies reported between the fathers and mothers in families with disabled children, reflecting their lower levels of agreement regarding family opportunities and coping (Margalit & Ankonina, 1991). These discrepancies were accentuated by the high agreement these mothers and fathers evidenced with one another with respect to the severity of their disabled child's maladjustment.

The finding of less involvement in activities leading to personal growth called for further study. In order to clarify whether the limited parental capacity to invest in their own personal growth resulted from their lower time, energy, and financial resources or from a subjective feeling of lower coherence, parents of disabled children were investigated in the Israeli kibbutz environment (Margalit, Leyser, Ankonina, & Avraham, 1991). The kibbutz society attempts to meet all of its members' individualized needs (such as food, lodging, medical care, recreation, and education), thus providing parents with the increased objective resources necessary for raising their disabled children. The severe demands on these objective resources due to the disabled child's special needs have often been attributed with causing stressful feelings.

These unique research comparisons revealed that parents of disabled children in the kibbutz expressed a similarly low personal sense of coherence to that of parents with disabled children in the city. In addition, parents with disabled children in the kibbutz and in the city alike reported similar family climate patterns. Their families were seen as less supportive and cohesive and as providing their members with fewer opportunities for personal growth in intellectual and cultural areas. This research study substantiated the impact of the subjective distress on families with a disabled child, despite differences in objective ecological conditions. Even when all of the increased coping needs were fulfilled through systemic support, materialistic provisions did not help to relieve the parental stress. In view of these and similar findings, recent research interest has been focused on the various means for increasing resilience and effective coping within the family system in contrast with factors within the family's distressful reality that contribute to loneliness feelings.

Family functioning style

Family strengths are considered to be the competencies and capabilities, among both individual family members and the family unit, which are used to promote the family's effective functioning in response to crises and stress, using Garmezy's (1983) emphasis on the importance of resilience and stress-resistance constructs. Family functioning style is the end-product of the interactions between the family's subjective definitions of their stressors and of the severity of the child's handicapping condition; the availability of resources to meet the greater needs; and the quality and efficiency of the coping strategies employed to introduce changes and re-organize the family's functioning (McCubbin & Patterson, 1983).

The study of family ecology within a family strengths model (Dunst, Trivette, & Deal, 1988) assumes that each family is characterized by various types of strengths and competencies that systematically define the style in which it affects the growth, socialization, and maturation of its members. All families have strengths that constitute valuable resources. By recognizing their presence and employing family strengths as one way of meeting needs, the resources that make the family work well are built upon, further empowering the family as a stronger unit that is more capable of negotiating the developmental tasks of its members. The conceptualization of family functioning style implies a unique, systemic (interpersonal and intrafamilial) manner of dealing with life events, including crises, and of meeting the needs and promoting the growth and development of individual family members.

The family functioning approach (Deal, Trivette, & Dunst, 1988; Trivette, Dunst, Deal, Hamer, & Propst, 1990) focused interest on identifying family strengths within the major patterns of functioning among strong, well-adjusted families. Within this model, major qualities of strong family systems were proposed, with the understanding that no one family would be expected to display all of these qualities. Instead, these qualities were considered dynamic, interrelated, and interactive, emphasizing the importance of studying family clusters and patterns.

Family strengths were designated by the following five major areas of functioning:

1 *Commitment* as the family members' investment of resources to promote the growth and well-being of the family members as well as the family unit.

2 *Cohesion* to support the needs of individual members within the system and the needs of the family system as a unit in order to enhance the members' growth.

3 *Competence* as demonstrated by appreciation for the things that the family members do well.

4 *Communication* as an information-sharing ability that fosters positive interactions among the family members.

5 *Coping* as a means of resource mobilization that includes various coping strategies to encourage effective problem solving, positive adjustment to life events, flexibility and adaptability in roles and resource allocation, and achieving a balance between intra- and extra-family resources for meeting needs.

Comparisons were conducted between the family functioning levels reported by parents of lonely and non-lonely adolescents (Efrati, 1993). The study revealed that the parents of the lonely youngsters viewed their family members as less competent and communicative. In addition, their family systems were perceived as less cohesive and committed and as demonstrating lower levels of coping.

Strong family typology

In an attempt to identify typologies of strength-oriented family functioning evaluated by parents and to examine its relations to adolescents' self-reported social and behavioral adjustment, 489 parental couples (fathers and mothers) and their adolescent children (248 male and 241 female students, aged 12 to 17 years; $M = 14.58$, $SD = 1.69$) were studied (Margalit, 1992). Cluster analysis on the basis of similarity over the parentally reported five family strengths yielded four family subtypes, as presented on Figure 3.1: strong, coping-oriented, strong identity-oriented, and least functioning.

Group A: Strong families (184 families - 37.6% of the sample). These fathers and mothers viewed their families as the most emphasizing and supporting of all five areas of family strengths, and as functioning at the highest level in all five areas of family functioning. These parents expressed high levels of commitment to the family system, felt that the family members were close to one another, with clear communication, and were also competent and able to cope with their difficulties. The adolescents exhibited less maladjustment, had better social skills, and felt less lonely.

Group B: Coping-oriented families (226 families - 46.2% of the sample). These parents viewed their families as highly emphasizing coping strategies. The adolescents reported intermediate levels of maladjustment, social skills, and loneliness.

Group C: Strong Identity-oriented families (42 families - 8.6% of the sample). These fathers and mothers viewed their families as emphasizing family identity aspects such as commitment and cohesiveness within the family system at high levels similar to Group A. These adolescents in many ways functioned similarly to the strongest families.

Group D: Least functioning families (37 families - 7.6% of the sample). These fathers and mothers viewed their families as the most poorly functioning families. Parents reported their family members to be the least competent, cohesive, or committed to the family affairs. Their children felt more lonely, had lower social skills, and showed more expressions of maladaptive behavior.

These data indicate the need to look more closely at the differential role of cohesion and commitment within the family climate as promoters of adolescents' social and behavioral adjustment. In homes that are committed and supportive of family members' individual needs, emphasizing communication and reinforcing their sense of competence, youngsters are aware of the family's support, develop better social skills, and even feel less lonely.

In order to fully understand the interrelations between aspects of the family environment and children's loneliness, parents' attitudes toward their children's lonely feelings and social functioning need to be explored.

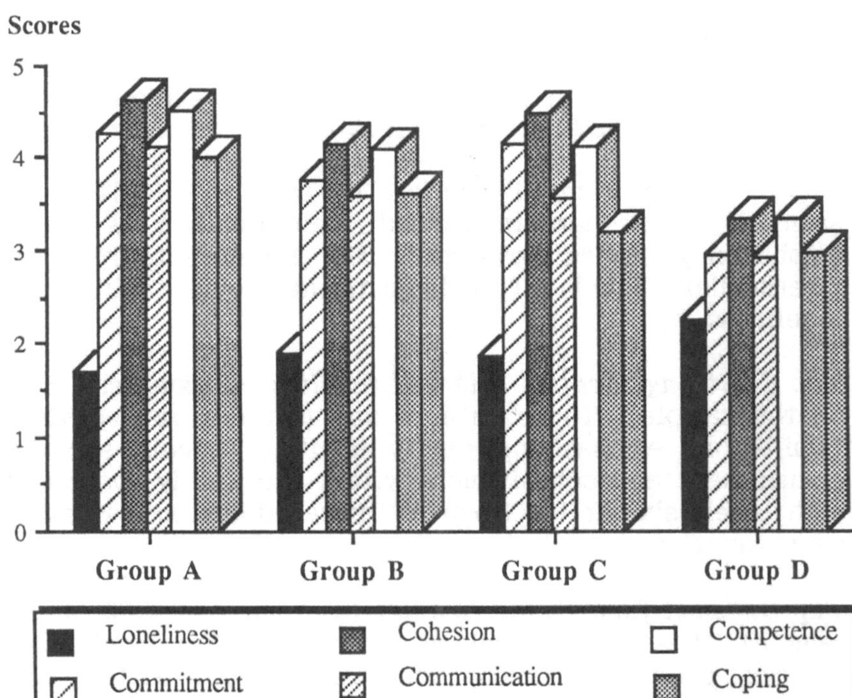

Figure 3.1 Four family functioning subgroups and children's adjustment

Loneliness and parental attitudes

Children with disabilities often experience academic and social difficulties, yet their learning problems are more often recognized and accepted than are their interpersonal ones. Many parents are willing to provide or search for the academic assistance that their children need. However, they often feel unprepared when facing children's complaints regarding their lack of friends and social isolation. The following case-study exemplifies this situation.

> *Dan, a 9-year-old boy with mild mental retardation, refused to go to school one morning following a weekend. His working mother was tense and confused. She did not have time for elaborated arguments, since she had to be at her office for an important meeting. When she tried to force him to go, he began crying and said, "It doesn't make any difference if I stay home or go to school. In any case, I'll be alone! I don't have any friends, or anybody to talk to or play with." When his mother tried to tell her son that when she was a little girl, she did not have many friends either, Dan told her through his tears, "But it's not the same! Everyone knows how dumb I am, and they all laugh at me."*
>
> *That day Dan's mother stayed home with her son and contacted his teacher. Annoyed, she heard the teacher supporting Dan's perceptions of social isolation and alienation, even with the other handicapped children in his self-contained special class. The teacher insisted that she felt resourceful only in academic subjects and rather helpless when it came to social attitudes. When the mother inquired why her son was so lonely, when he was in a class with other children who were also functioning at a similar academic level, the teacher replied sadly, "They are all very lonely."*

This description reflects the feelings of helplessness of parents and teachers when confronted with expressions of children's loneliness. Ladd (1988) found that the interest revealed by parents of preschoolers in their children's social interactions and friendships was rather limited, especially in comparison to the major emphasis placed on their academic performance. This finding can be understood not only as a manifestation of the priority given to the important task of learning during childhood, but also as an expression of parents' helplessness feelings. When children fail to learn the alphabet or numbers, particularly during preschool and the early grades of schooling, it seems rather clear what can be done to help them. However, parents feel that they do not know how to assist their children when they face social difficulties, given that the causes of the problems are often attributed to other children and seem beyond their control. They feel that they cannot change other children's attitudes and feelings toward their own children. Parents feel more effective at helping children with academic rather than social tasks or peer relations. Parental interest and involvement in their children's social functioning and difficulties with peers has only recently become the subject of research. Parents have begun to articulate their views regarding the importance of enhancing the social competence of their children, with the goal of increasing not only academic and life skills but also friendships (Hamre-Nietupski, Nietupski, & Strathe, 1992).

In an attempt to assess parental views regarding their children's loneliness and social competence, 40 boys with learning disabilities and their mothers and teachers were compared to matched groups without disabilities (Unger, 1992). The learning disabled boys were viewed as more lonely than the nondisabled group, with mothers and children appraising similarly the loneliness levels for both groups of boys. In addition, the correlations between mothers and their sons were significant only for the disabled group ($r = .44$). Teachers of both groups of students viewed the youngsters as much more lonely than did the children themselves or the mothers. No significant correlations were found between teachers and students in either group, yet the correlations between teachers and mothers for the disabled group were significant ($r = .41$). It was also found that loneliness feelings as rated by mothers were predicted by their assessment of the boys' behavior difficulties and social skills. This pioneer study on perceptions of children's loneliness by the significant adults in their lives pinpoints attention onto mothers of learning disabled children as judging the child's social situation similarly to the child's self-report. (Teachers' attitudes and impact will be more fully explored in Chapter 4.) These shared perceptions between mothers and learning disabled children represent another aspect of the transactional model. The following case-study presents an example of parents' empathetic approach to their children's experience of loneliness.

> *Sharon's learning disabled daughter was extremely depressed. Her mother contacted the school counselor, saying that both she and her daughter could hear the neighbors' children visiting one another and spending time together, while nobody called her daughter. When Sharon observed her daughter watching TV for hours on end without any interest, she visualized all of her own lonely childhood experiences. "It almost paralyzes you to see all your early difficulties, that were almost forgotten as an adult, coming back much more powerfully and painfully."*

This mother's empathy with her daughter's loneliness and her own memories of childhood social isolation resulted in Sharon viewing her daughter's social difficulties as a major source of the mother's stress and feelings of helplessness. It is not surprising that children's loneliness may be considered a source of parental distress and helplessness, yet the parents' own personal history of social relations or alienation may affect their reactions and coping strategies. As a group, higher levels of loneliness were reported for parents with disabled children, such as mothers with learning disabled children (Hofmann, 1983) and mothers whose children had chronic illnesses (Florian & Krulik, 1991). In view of the fact that parents' own loneliness experiences may affect their attitudes towards their children's loneliness reports, any intervention should consider parental involvement and the bidirectional influence of expressions of sadness and pain.

Conclusions

Children's loneliness was presented in this chapter as related to various aspects within the family environment. The study of loneliness as an interplay between situations and personal characteristics pointed attention at both individual and systemic experiences as joint determinants of the loneliness experience (Large, 1989). Different approaches have similarly considered the nature of parent-child interactions to be the root of social competence, providing children with the confidence, knowledge, and experience that will serve as the basis for later social growth and peer relations. The present paradigm attempted to identify those factors which may either exacerbate parental feelings of distress and children's social difficulties or may serve a stress-resistance role in buffering stressful realities and in empowering parental active coping and children's social growth.

The systemic approach in family studies attempted to identify critical elements and processes that are locked together in promoting the children's growth and affecting their abilities to develop meaningful and satisfying social interrelations. Parent-child interactions were considered the end product of parental characteristics including their reactions to disability-related stress, children's characteristics including their specific needs, and family resources including functioning style. Parents' sense of coherence, the family's strengths and capacity for successful adjustment, and parental beliefs, attitudes, and coping abilities all join together in presenting disabled children with an environment that may either promote their capacity to form companionship and intimacy or else support their isolation and alienation. Recent research directed toward a reconceptualization of the attachment construct, through a clarification of the link between parent-child interrelations and later loneliness and social competence, has highlighted the process as a dynamic and prolonged one. Children were found to be continually renegotiating the balance between being connected to others and being independent and autonomous as they entered new developmental phases.

Children's disabilities introduce changes into both the world of family and the world of peers. The processes within the family environment can be treated as the roots for social growth, but also as an ongoing force shaping the child's social experiences. The peer world, with its companionship relations and accepting/rejecting attitudes, can be considered as the critical social environment for experimenting with social skills and for experiencing friendship and loneliness.

4 Peer Relations and Children's Friendships

The study of relations not only in the family system but also in the peer environment provides important information for the understanding of children's loneliness. Why do some children become well-liked or accepted by peers, whereas others are rejected or ignored? Why do some of these rejected children feel lonely, whereas others do not? Questions like these, dealing with the complexity of peer relations, have recently become the focus of research interest. A great deal of consensus already exists concerning the perceived benefits of early and different patterns of relations, not only with family members but also with peers, for the development of satisfying social competence throughout life (Rubin, 1985; Rubin & Mills, 1988). During childhood, individuals learn a wide variety of social behaviors and responses, including prosocial and aggressive acts, sex roles, and emotional reactions (Ladd, 1988). Peers may serve as effective models and reinforcers of socially appropriate behaviors and may help in reducing children's distress in unfamiliar and threatening situations; in addition, spending time with peers may provide children with unique opportunities to discuss feelings, expand thought processes and knowledge, and experiment with age-related task performance and social roles (Ladd, 1988).

Children with disabilities from the earliest stages of socialization were observed spending more time alone than did normally developing children (Kopp, Baker, & Brown, 1992). As early as age three, children with developmental delays revealed nonverbal cues as to their inability or unwillingness to be a play partner. These young children demonstrated more periods when uninvolved in play or unoccupied and also evidenced more regressive and disruptive entry behaviors. Time alone represents missed opportunities to experiment with social interactions, and regressive conduct can be alienating for peers.

Poor peer relations may be treated both as an index of adjustment problems and as a contributor to future difficulties. Without entering into the ongoing debate about the etiology of emotional disorders as conceptualized by different theoretical approaches, poor peer relations are usually viewed either as an early manifestation of emotional difficulties or as a factor leading to such disorders if left untreated (Rubin & Mills, 1988). Longitudinal data have indicated that rejection by peers during childhood may be considered a high risk factor for later antisocial behavior, school dropout, and poor mental health (Parker & Asher, 1987). Regardless of whether poor peer relations are a driving force in development or merely a barometer of general psychological distress and adjustment (Rubin & Mills, 1988), children with social dysfunction are likely to be at risk for some form of psychological maladjustment requiring early identification and individualized intervention (Ladd, 1988).

Much research on social relations has been focused on two specific types of peer relationships among children:

1 Acceptance and status in peer groups
2 Friendships

Social status, in terms of acceptance and popularity, and friendships, in terms of the size and quality of intimate relations, represent distinct developmental functions that are not strongly correlated and that predict different outcomes (Berndt, 1990). The concept of peer status refers to the child's interrelations with all of the group, whereas the concept of friendship refers to a specific relationship between children's dyads.

Social status: Acceptance and rejection

Even as early as the preschool stage, children become organized into subgroups of youngsters who prefer each other's company or who share common characteristics or interests. Some children find themselves in a larger peer group only when starting preschool, whereas others already have their first experience with peer groups at very early stages of development, either at home or in the neighborhood (Ellis,

Rogoff, & Cromer, 1981; Ladd, Hart, & Wadsworth, 1988). The concept of peer status refers to a group's attitudes toward or acceptance of a child. Peer status or acceptance is often defined as the degree to which the child is liked or disliked by group members (Ladd, 1988). Likability may be related to cooperative relations for performing a specific task like preparing a school project in a small working group or playing a game. Each group has one or several leaders and many followers, and children as early as four years of age were able to discriminate stable levels of likability among peers and to identify children who possess different levels of social status.

Although a number of sociometric procedures have been employed in social research, peer status is typically assessed by asking the members of a particular group (e.g., the classroom) to either rate or nominate each other in terms of perceived likability (e.g., "Whom do you like to play with? Who would you like to invite to your party? With whom do you not like planning a task?"). The averaged ratings or the number of positive and/or negative nominations received from peers are used to define and categorize the children's status within the group. Five different status classifications have been defined by research (Coie, Dodge, & Coppotelli, 1982):

1. *Popular.* Children who receive many positive nominations from peers and only a few negative nominations are considered liked by peers.

2. *Rejected.* Children who receive few positive nominations and many negative nominations are considered disliked.

3. *Neglected.* Children who tend to be overlooked receive few nominations (either positive or negative) from peers.

4. *Controversial.* These are children who are well-liked by many peers but also very disliked by many peers.

5. *Average.* Children who receive roughly equal numbers of positive and negative nominations are considered liked and/or disliked by peers but not to an extreme in either direction.

Several longitudinal studies revealed that these status definitions remain relatively stable throughout the school years

(Cillessen, Van Lieshout, & Haselager, 1992; Coie & Dodge, 1983; Ladd, 1988) and that low peer status in childhood is an important antecedent of later adjustment problems (Parker & Asher, 1987).

Students with disabilities have been often considered to be a population at high risk for peer rejection. Many learning disabled students receive low social ratings from peers, are defined as having a low social status, and are identified as rejected or isolated in their classrooms (Bruininks, 1978; Bryan, 1974; Bryan & Bryan, 1978; Perlmutter, Crocker, Cordray, & Garstecki, 1983; Stone & LaGreca, 1990). Even when learning disabled children were rated by their own learning disabled peers within self-contained educational systems, their acceptance scores were lower than those of nondisabled children who were rated by their nondisabled peers (Margalit & Ben-Dov, 1992). The social dissatisfaction of learning disabled students was expressed by the lower sociometric scores that these children gave their disabled peers, highlighting their judgments of peers as less desirable socially. In a recent comprehensive survey, Pearl (1992) reported on findings from a vast database of research, clearly suggesting that learning disabled students be treated as a high risk group for current and future social rejections and alienation. Nevertheless, she pointed out that not all learning disabled students were found to be rejected, and that some studies (Sabornie & Kauffman, 1986; Sabornie, Marshall, & Ellis, 1988) failed to find significant differences regarding social status between students with learning disabilities and nonhandicapped students.

In Stone and LaGreca's (1990) research, 75% of the children with learning disabilities fell into one of the low status groups, where they were represented almost equally in the rejected and neglected categories. These findings suggested that learning disabled children who experience peer problems may actually consist of two distinct subgroups: some of whom experience active peer rejection and others who are more likely to be ignored by their classmates. Within this learning disabled sample, the rejected children were found to be more likely to demonstrate aggressive and disruptive behavior, whereas the neglected children were more likely to be shy and withdrawn and to experience social anxiety. Low peer ratings have also been found for children with behavior difficulties such as aggressiveness and disruptiveness at different ages, from preschoolers to adolescents (Asher, Parkhurst, Hymel, &

Williams, 1990; Cramer & Skidd, 1992; Parkhurst & Asher, 1992; Sabornie, Marshall, & Ellis, 1988).

On the basis of current research, peer rejection can be viewed as an important index to be assessed during childhood, necessitating a better understanding of the phenomenon. Coie's (1990) model was developed in order to clarify how peer rejection becomes established and maintains itself through children's developmental stages.

Peer rejection model

Coie's (1990) model of peer rejection is based on the assumption that social behavior is the primary cause for rejection by peers. Although non-behavioral factors such as appearance, academic achievement, disabilities, and athletic competence also have an important impact on peers' evaluations, the proposed model assumes that children dislike certain peers not because they are deficient in some critical areas, but because of the way in which they interact with peers. According to Coie, the social difficulties of rejected children seem to result from the way they interpret specific social situations and from their emotional reactions and acquired strategies for dealing with these situations.

Coie posited that these social behavior patterns, affective reactions, and interpretations of situations emerge out of the child's socialization history. Individual differences such as temperament, abilities, and disabilities are significant determinants of subsequent social functioning; and environmental variables such as differences in parental effectiveness may also play a role. However, the unique patterns of the child's reactions to specific social interactions is largely shaped by the history of the child's interactions with parent figures, siblings, and peers. Inherited and ecological predispositional factors may have greater impact on children's behaviors at times, such as in some cases where children, because of biologically-linked attributes, may be more at risk for triggering adverse or exaggerated responses from social figures in their environment; or where some parents may be less effective at handling their infant, regardless of whether the child has a placid or an irritable temperament. Yet this model primarily emphasizes the transactional nature of relations and activities: For example, a highly punitive but inconsistent parent will have a deleterious effect on most children, yet the behavior of a hyperactive child may succeed in initiating even more emotional reactions from this parent.

Peer interactions related to acceptance and rejection may be seen as resembling the pattern of interactions within the family. In family interactions, the child both affects and is affected by other family members, getting reinforcement for some reactions and punishment for others, and thereby learning social behavior that will affect the child's future social status. In addition, family climate in general and parental attitudes and behaviors in particular serve as models for interpersonal behavior. In the peer group, children affect and are affected by other children, receiving the group's accepting or rejecting attitudes and behaviors as a consequence of their own activities. Thus, the child's individual social history leads to difficulties in coping with specific types of interpersonal events not only in the family context. These difficulties over time continue to formulate the basis for future social problems in other contextual environments such as the peer group.

Coie proposed that the two sources of peer rejection -- the behavior of the children and the dynamics of the group -- interact differently at various stages in the development of social rejection. The process of acquiring social status in the peer group was conceptualized as having different dynamics than the process of maintaining a stable identity as a rejected child. At the stage of entry into peer interactions, the most important determinant seems to be the child's behavior, which is evaluated by the peers and compared to an expected standard; the peer dynamic in the group has been considered only secondary and less significant in explaining the initial stages of the rejection process. However, the model posits that after the children have gained a reputation as rejected and disliked by a significant number of peers, the group dynamic becomes more important. At this stage, group opinion may be conceptualized as affecting the individual group members in two ways: directly -- affecting the behavior of rejected children, who adjust their behavior to subjective expectations and interpretations, and indirectly -- affecting the perceptions, cognitions, and behaviors of the group members. As the children experience rejection, their feelings about themselves change, decreasing their sense of social confidence and security.

Indirect causal effects on the future adjustment of these children have been attributed to sustained peer rejection. The consistent experience of rejection may affect their cognitive processes, affective responses, and behavior. They may develop inadequate social skills for future stressful events and may have a limited social support network during the adolescent phase, along with fewer opportunities to model adaptive behavior styles and to develop successful coping strategies.

Explanations vary for the predictive efficacy of early peer status. Ladd (1988) stated that low peer acceptance (i.e., rejection) has debilitating effects on children's personal and interpersonal development, inhibiting children's social learning (e.g., exclusion from group activities may enable them to learn fewer social skills) and reducing their sense of belonging and self-esteem. A survey of longitudinal studies (Asher & Renshaw, 1981; Asher, Hymel, & Renshaw, 1984; Asher & Wheeler, 1985; Ladd, 1988; Wheeler & Ladd, 1982) revealed that once children become disliked, they face a growing difficulty in finding steady play partners. They have limited opportunities to interact with popular children, tending to interact mostly with peers who have the same status, and in general spending more time alone or interacting in small groups with younger and/or unpopular companions. Rejected children were found to have less social support not only from peer groups but also from teachers. They were more lonely, less self-confident, and more likely to be depressed.

In an attempt to analyze the interactional style of rejected children, research has investigated the different stages of their social behavior. These youngsters were found to be less effective and less successful even in initiating interactions and in their entry behavior into a group (Putallaz & Wasserman, 1990). Observations during interactions revealed that the rejected children failed to remain engaged with other children for long periods, but rather moved from interaction to interaction more frequently than did the other children (Ladd, 1983). The analysis provided support for the tenet that the sources of social problems rest not only in the rejected individuals themselves but also in their peers' behavior style toward them. In line with the transactional model of behavior, it was found that rejected children were the recipients of fewer positive initiations and more negative interactions from their peers (Dodge, 1983).

Developmental perspectives on peer rejection

Within the research base on peer relations, the developmental dimension has been studied with the goal of identifying patterns that may enhance understanding of the processes and factors involved in social status over time. Research studies conducted with different groups have demonstrated the developmental relations to factors leading to peer acceptance and rejection.

Preschool level

Peer acceptance and rejection have been assessed as early as the preschool developmental stage. Coie, Dodge, and Kupersmidt's (1990) comprehensive survey of social status research concluded that data from preschool peers, teachers, and observers are surprisingly unidimensional, presenting a consistent social reality with respect to the correlates of high status or acceptance among preschool children. High status preschool children were described as helpful and considerate of others and as following rules, particularly the rules for peer interaction. They were described as more engaged in positive peer interaction.

Wasik (1987) administered peer assessments to 52 kindergarten children at several intervals and found that being cooperative within the children's group was positively and consistently related to social preferences. Conversely, starting fights and being disruptive was consistently negatively related to social preference. Cramer and Skidd (1992) emphasized in their research the importance of sex-stereotyped styles of behavior. It seems that children whose style of social interaction was characteristically sex-stereotyped received more positive feedback from peers, and in turn demonstrated a greater sense of self-worth than did children whose style of interaction was less sex-stereotyped. Withdrawing and retreating behaviors were negatively related to self-worth and peer acceptance for both boys and girls. However, a stronger relationship appeared in boys than in girls between the use of gender-stereotyped behaviors and a sense of peer acceptance and self-worth, results that are consistent with the greater pressure on boys to conform to sex-stereotyped behaviors and to avoid behaviors that contradict sex-role stereotypes (Maccoby & Jacklin, 1980).

In the search for predictors of likability within the preschool age group, the importance of the affective domain was recognized, and the powerful role of emotions as intrapersonal and interpersonal regulators of behaviors was the focus of study (Denham, McKinley, Couchoud, & Holt, 1990). Research reported that preschool peers found it easier and more pleasant to interact with emotionally positive children, rating happy children as more popular, whereas angrier children were rated as less likeable (Rubin & Clark, 1983). Denham, McKinley, Couchoud, and Holt (1990) demonstrated in their study that those children who were able to control their own negative emotions were viewed as generally feeling happy and reacting positively to peers and also were judged by peers as more likeable. Children who showed predominantly negative emotions, whether expressing sad, angry, or hurt moods, also showed varying deficits in social understanding and/or prosocial domains and were more rejected. These findings seem to indicate that prosocial and nonaggressive behaviors such as friendliness, nurturance, and altruism, rather than aggression or preoccupation with one's own distress, develop rather early as responses to others' emotional displays. Children who failed to develop these responses appeared to be at risk of being disliked (Denham, McKinley, Couchoud, & Holt, 1990). However detailed examination revealed that just being a "smiler" did not guarantee positive peer ratings for the child. Positive expressions of affect without adequate prosocial skills did not lead to social acceptance. Likability levels at the preschool stage were found to be fairly stable and to differentiate well between those children who were more adept at understanding emotional situations (i.e., the more prosocial and popular children) and those who were less proficient (i.e., the rejected ones) (Denham, McKinley, Couchoud, & Holt, 1990). Children with disabilities as a group, even at the preschool age, received significantly lower peer ratings from both same-age and younger developmentally matched children without disabilities (Guralnick & Groom, 1987). It seems that they were identified as less accepted by peers from their earliest experiences in the educational system (Vaughn & Hogan, 1990; Vaughn, Hogan, Kouzekanani, & Shapiro, 1990).

Elementary school level

During elementary school, the sociometric status of children is already well established. The findings for 8-12 year olds were consistent with those of the younger children, with the exception that greater emphasis was placed on the athletic and academic competence of popular children. Peer reports of well-liked individuals revealed that this emphasis on the competence aspects was found to continue through the adolescent stage.

Rejected elementary school children seem to experience

dissatisfaction from their social relations (Asher, Parkhurst, Hymel, & Williams, 1990). Feeling disliked by the majority of children in their class transforms their daily social climate into a negative one. It should be clearly stated that consistent evidence exists demonstrating that peer relations do matter to rejected children, who may be expected to experience frustrations, dissatisfaction, and negative emotional consequences. In studies of third through sixth graders (Asher, Hymel, & Renshaw, 1984; Asher, Parkhurst, Hymel, & Williams, 1990), the poorly accepted children tended to express higher levels of loneliness feelings than did their better accepted peers. The children's self-reported loneliness and social dissatisfaction score was negatively and significantly related to their peer acceptance as measured by sociometric ratings. Yet, the moderate magnitude of the correlations obtained reflects the fact that not all unpopular children report feeling lonely and that some popular children do feel lonely, indicating the existence of subgroups and of factors (such as having a good friend) that mediate the loneliness experience.

Middle and high school levels

Parkhurst and Asher (1992) examined peer relations in middle school and found considerable continuity with the results from studies of younger children. The profile of the popular middle school student was similar to that of the popular elementary school student: low on aggressiveness and disruptiveness, average on assertive dimensions, and perceived by peers as cooperative and trustworthy. As among the younger samples, rejected status was associated with aggressiveness and disruptiveness and with a lack of prosocial qualities. Research surveys on rejection and peer status in adolescence stressed the predominance of isolation and emotionality during this period, whereas aggression as a predictive factor decreased in importance (Kupersmidt, Coie, & Dodge, 1990).

Children with disabilities were considered a high risk group for experiencing rejection throughout the different age stages of their educational experience. Their lower levels of peer acceptance reflect their characteristics and behavior, resulting in patterns of peer interaction that lead to rejection. However, not all of the disabled children experience a high level of loneliness, focusing attention on factors that mediate the peer rejection, such as companionship and friendship. In addition, for some children, rejection is limited to certain peer contexts or age groups, whereas other children exhibit a persistent social experience of rejection. The duration and relative intensity of peer rejection should be studied within the developmental perspective in order to further clarify predictive issues.

Friendship relations

Friendships are manifested through mutual interests and preferences, attraction, closeness, intimacy, and the extent to which these perceptions are stable and shared by both members of the dyads. Even at the preschool stage, children can identify other children as "friends," gradually developing stable associations with play companions. Although friendship is a private experience that can best be described through self-reports, often these relations become recognized by teachers, parents, and even other children. In social research, information on stable associations with specific peers has been provided by children with and without disabilities and by the significant adults in their environments. Observations of children's interactions during experimental task performance indicated that they interact differently with friends than with strangers, showing greater mutuality with friends (Coie, 1990; Waas & Honer, 1990). Students with disruptive behavior and students with withdrawn behavior were less competent, experiencing lower levels of the mutuality, responsiveness, and positive behaviors that characterize friendship relations (Panella & Henggeler, 1986).

Children's friendships were shown to negatively predict feelings of loneliness regardless of peer acceptance levels. Children without best friends demonstrated more loneliness than did children with best friends. Among individuals with developmental disabilities, those who reported not having a friend described themselves more negatively than did those with friends (Clegg & Standen, 1991). However, the factors that enable a child to establish and maintain friendships appear to differ from the factors leading to peer acceptance (Rizzo, 1988). The low correlations between social status and measures of friendship pinpointed attention to the finding that some low status children, who are rated overall as poorly accepted by their peer groups, do have best friends. Furthermore, according to mutual nominations, only about two-thirds of highly accepted children have good friends (Parker & Asher, in press). These results suggest that the "good friend" situation may have potential as a major predictor of loneliness and as a critical issue in the life of disabled and nondisabled children alike.

In an attempt to clarify the role of friendship in predicting feelings of loneliness (Parker & Asher, in press), two main elements of friendship need to be examined: the quantity of good friends and the quality of friendship relations. The first element, children's quantitative participation in friendship bonding or the size of the social network, can be evaluated outside the school setting by children's self-reports and within schools by identifying reciprocal choices among the patterns of nominations children give in response to questions about who are their best friends. Research has shown that loneliness is linked to the quantity of one's social interactions, with lonely individuals indicating that they have less friends, spend more time alone, and are engaged in fewer social activities than non-lonely individuals.

The second element, quality of friendship, is always the product of complex interactions between the personal characteristics of the individual and his/her partner, and the context or history of the relationships. Friendship has emergent subjective properties such as role expectations and obligations that may affect these individual characteristics.

Size of social network

Using a simplistic approach, the process of estimating an individual's number of friends or social network size does not seem complicated and can be achieved by asking children to name their best friends and calculating the quantity measure on the basis of the number of nominated peers. However, these measures prove less consistent than expected, and the size of the social network is often difficult to estimate, due to children's tendencies to have differing and in some cases inconsistent relationship styles. The term "friend" seems to be defined dissimilarly by different children at separate times, ranging from close, intimate friends to more superficial partnerships aimed at joint task performance, or even to fellow members of a larger network such as the classroom, thus providing an inconsistent picture, reflecting individualistic interpretations of the construct. When asked how many friends they have, or to name their best friends, different children will refer to various social networks of different sizes as related to their personal conception of "good" friendships. However, several generalizations can be concluded.

For preschool children, the quantity of friendships was considered important. It was reported that young children who have many friends often spend more time interacting with those friends and comparatively less time in solitary play or with adults such as teachers, in comparison to children with few friends (Rizzo, 1988). Rizzo's study suggested that one of the reasons for young children's engagement in nonsocial behavior is a relatively fewer number of friends with whom to play. Having many friends may help the process of entrance into peer play and acceptance by the group.

The number of different peers seen by children on a regular basis (who may be identified as friends without entering into the complex question of the qualitative meaning of friendship) has been found to increase with age. On the average, preschool children had regular contacts with three to four children, whereas children at the beginning of elementary school regularly met with five to six peers (Ladd, 1988). Ladd described the tendency for children's peer networks to become more homogeneous over time with respect to age and gender. As children grow older, more of their companions are of the same age and sex. In addition, the duration of friendships has been found to be related to developmental stage. When asked how long specific children have been their friends, children revealed that friendships generally tend to be relatively stable and to increase in duration with age. Ladd and Emerson (1984) reported that first graders had known their friends for an average of 3.6 months, whereas fourth graders described a more extended period of relations -- an average of 7.2 months.

Gender differences have also been shown regarding the number of friendships. Boys and girls differ in terms of the range or number of different peers with whom they have contacts in their peer groups. Boys typically have a broader range of peers with whom they have more contacts. Girls tend to have fewer friends, to make friendships more slowly, and to differentiate between friends and acquaintances more clearly (Ladd, 1988). In addition, both boys and girls were found to interact with a large range of peers at the beginning of the school year but to eventually focus most of their contacts on a few consistent companions.

Clear individual differences are evident in the number of friends among children. Some have many friends, whereas some have a few or none at all. The number of friends is related both to situational factors (e.g., classroom climate) and personal factors (e.g., a preference for a smaller number of friends). Rizzo (1988) investigated the size of the social network (i.e., existing friendships) among children rated as rejected, average, and popular. Virtually all children had at least one friend, highlighting that even rejected children are not friendless.

Quantity of friends among disabled children

Studies have investigated friendships among children with a variety of disabling conditions. In a study of 40 boys with learning disabilities in grades 6 to 8 (mean age = 13.30, SD = 1.16), only three children (7.5%) reported that they did not have any friends, and an additional three reported having only one friend (Unger, 1992). The number of friends ranged from none to nine, but 70% of the sample (28 children) reported having two to five friends, and only nine children had more than five friends. The children met most of these friends at school in the morning (30 children - 75%) and in their neighborhoods during afternoons and weekends (27 children - 67.5%).

Similar results were reported in Zehavi's (1992) study, in which two age groups of mainstreamed learning disabled students were investigated: the younger group consisted of 20 students in grades 2 to 4, and the older group consisted of 20 students in grades 6 to 8. The potential number of friends ranged from none to nine, yet all of the children reported having at least one friend, and most children (61.5%) had two to five friends. Most friends were schoolmates (91.4%), but 28 children also met friends in their neighborhood (80%). The comparison between the number of friends in the two different age groups revealed that the older children had a significantly larger network of friends (younger group: M = 3.42, SD = 1.31; older group: M = 5.38, SD = 2.02). The correlation between the number of friends and self-reported loneliness was negative and significant but low for both age groups (r = -.33).

In a study of 157 adolescents from special education settings with an age range of 11 to 16 years, similar findings were demonstrated (Margalit, 1993a). This sample consisted of 116 students with behavior disorders (ages: M = 13.27; SD = 1.53) and 41 students with learning disabilities (ages: M = 11.94, SD = 1.07). The number of friends ranged from none to nine. Eight adolescents with behavior disorders (6.9%) reported not having any friends, and 63 behavior disordered students (54.3%) and 28 learning disabled students (68.3%) reported having two to four friends. No significant differences in the number of friends were found between the two groups of special education students in the sample. The mean number of friends was 3.53 (*SD* = 2.30) for the group with behavior disorders and 3.59 (*SD* = 1.61) for the second group. The correlation for both groups between number of friends and self-reported feelings of loneliness was negative and significant but low ($r = -.28$), suggesting the importance of a focus on the quality of friendship for understanding its role.

Friendship quality

In contrast to research linking loneliness to the quantity of one's social interactions, other investigations indicate that the quality of social interactions has more influence on feelings of loneliness (Chelune, Sultan, & Williams, 1980; Jones, 1981). This approach emphasizes not the number of social interactions or their frequency, but their quality, focusing on the nature of interactions with friends and family. Similarly to the different relation provisions proposed by Josselson (1992), a good friend may provide the child with one or more of the following four provisions:

1 Help and support
2 Companionship and recreation
3 Intimate exchange
4 Validation of self-worth

Help and support

> *"A good friend is someone you can ask to help you. If I need a help, I can always ask him for it, and I don't have to be shy"* (Ron - a 15-year-old male student with learning disabilities).
>
> *"You can ask a friend for a favor without feeling embarrassed or uncomfortable, and she will do whatever it is you need, willingly and without a second thought"* (Sharon - a 17-year-old female adolescent with behavior disorders).

"Good friends help me with my studies and bring me homework when I'm sick" (Gila - a 12-year-old girl with learning disabilities).

"Good friends listen to me and help me find ways to solve my problems" (Gal - a 10-year-old boy with learning disabilities).

"They help me and protect me when I fight with other children" (Ran - a 15-year-old student with mild mental retardation).

This aspect of friendship deals with the provisions of assistance, help, and guidance when the need arises. It is related to providing materialistic resources and/or emotional support to one's friends. Learning disabled children viewed this aspect of friendship as most important, with more than half of the group studied expecting a good friend to provide them with help and support (Unger, 1992; Zehavi, 1992). During interviews (Margalit, 1993a) with children having different handicapping conditions, the friend's role as a source of help was described in similar proportions for two groups: 70 students with behavior disorders (60.34%) and 22 students with learning disabilities (53.65%) viewed this provision as important in their friends.

Companionship and recreation

"We go out a lot together, to parties, to see films, have a good time together, laugh together" (Yoav - a 12-year-old boy with behavior disorders).

"We stay together almost all day, having lots of fun together" (Avraham - a 10-year-old boy with learning disabilities).

"When I don't have anything to do and I'm bored, I can always call her or go over there and we play together. And especially, there's another thing -- we talk all the time on the telephone" (Miriam - an 8-year-old girl with attention deficit disorder).

"A good friend doesn't ever leave me alone. We hang around in school together, do our homework together, play during the afternoon. It's fun to spend time together with each other" (Orit - a 7-year-old girl with learning disabilities).

The friendship relationship provides children with opportunities for play, companionship, recreation, and the enjoyable use of time together. When asked to define what a friend is, most children with and without disabilities referred to leisure and recreation time in specific and nonspecific terms. A friend was described as someone with whom to spend time, to play different games, or even with whom to "hang around" without having any specific plans.

When interviewed, about half of children with learning disabilities described a friend as someone with whom they spend free time or have a good time (Unger, 1992; Zehavi, 1992). In Margalit's (1993a) study, a significant difference was found between the groups with learning disabilities and behavior disorders. More students with learning disabilities (51.21%) than students with behavior disorders (33.62%) viewed the friend's major role as a free time companion. In an attempt to avoid boredom and situations where they had nothing to do during afternoons or weekends, the role of the friend as a companion was highly valued.

Intimate exchange

> *"I tell her secrets, and she tells me, even about her family or about boys"* (Rina - a 9-year-old girl with behavior disorders).
>
> *"He listens to me, cares about me, and we tell one another everything. We can laugh together and tell secrets"* (Asaf - a 10-year-old boy with learning disabilities).
>
> *"A good friend is somebody who shares with me whatever happens to her, and we can talk about everything"* (Gila - a 12-year-old girl with behavior disorders).
>
> *"I trust him that he won't tell anybody else about my feelings. We talk about everything -- girls, parents, and school"* (Yaniv - a 14-year-old boy with learning disabilities).

A friend is a child with whom the relationship is characterized by the sharing of secrets and private concerns and by the disclosure of personal information and feelings. Only one child out of the forty children in the learning disabled group in Unger's (1992) study mentioned sharing feelings and thoughts as one of the characteristics of a friend. In Margalit's (1993a) study, 20 students (17.24%) in the behavior disordered sample and two students (5.30%) in the sample with learning disabilities mentioned this provision.

Validation of self-worth

> *"A good friend accepts me as I am, appreciates me and does not try to ridicule or change me"* (Sara - a 17-year-old girl with behavior disorders).
>
> *"It is important to me that my friend tells me what he thinks about me, without insulting me, and understands how I feel and what I do"* (Ronen - 12-year-old boy with learning disabilities).

Children find the friendship relationship important for learning to see themselves through comparisons with others, thus enhancing and validating self-worth. Adolescent students, for example, who viewed their friendships as more positive or supportive reported higher perceived social acceptance and higher general self-worth (Ladd, 1988). Students who viewed their friendships more negatively had lower perceptions of self-worth. This provision was not described by any of the special education groups (Margalit & Al-Yagon, in press; Unger, 1992; Zehavi, 1992).

Conflict resolution

In addition to the provisions offered by friendships, another dimension to be considered in evaluating the quality of friendship is through investigating the conflicts and disagreements between children -- the extent that the relationship is typified by arguments, quarrels, annoyance, and mistrust (Parker & Asher, in press). Conflicts often occur among children, and may be considered to represent different points of view, attitudes, and interests. Special attention should be focused on conflict resolution patterns -- the degree to which disagreements within the friendship relations are resolved, with an emphasis on their efficient and fair resolution. The types of conflicts that children experience, their affective impact, and the ease and readiness with which these conflicts are resolved therefore represent distinct dimensions worthy of investigation within the exploration of the quality of friendships.

Research on quality aspects

Parker and Asher's (in press) study examined gender differences regarding the quality of friendship relations and found that two dimensions did not differentiate between boys and girls: (a) conflict and betrayal and (b) companionship and recreational activities. However, girls did report higher levels than boys on the following friendship dimensions: (a) validation, (b) support and help, (c) conflict resolution, and (d) intimate exchange. These differences may stem from the different play styles and group structures of boys when compared to girls. Boys usually play in larger groups that are more hierarchically organized, and the relationships they develop tend to be less close. However, these recent findings call for more research.

In an attempt to validate the qualitative friendship experience, Parker and Asher (in press) compared the perceived characteristics of friendship relations between 133 pairs of best friends. They compared the perceptions of companionship as provided by dyads of friends and found that the correspondence between the two partners' ratings on the different aspects of the friendship relations ranged from higher correlations for aspects such as companionship and recreation (expressing a high level of agreement between dyads) to lower correlations regarding conflict resolution (indicating considerable differences). These results either represent real differences in the individuals' perceptions of experiences, or else signal that the dyads did not have shared expectations and understanding of the meaning of one another's behavior.

Individual patterns of friendship lead to different social provisions that can be expected to point to distinct personal needs. These differences make the evaluation of the value and level of companionship complicated, highlighting the need to interview children with disabilities in detail concerning their friendship relations. In addition, the findings linking friendship relations to self-perceptions such as self-worth should be treated within the concept of reciprocality. It is not clear whether lower self-worth leads to less satisfaction from various areas of functioning including friendship, or whether dissatisfying peer relations cause a lower sense of self-worth. The satisfaction and dissatisfaction from friendship relations focuses interest on the friendship-making process.

Friendship and status

How do children initially choose their friends? Children often select friends from the same or similar social status. Yet, friends are not chosen strictly on the basis of status: Some accepted children develop friendship relations with some rejected children. Neither is time spent with friends a valid differentiating measure: Accepted and rejected children were found to spend the same amount of time with their individual friends. The finding that rejected children sometimes do have friends who are not rejected, and that the investigation of time spent with different status children did not show differences, suggests that differences in social status do not translate in simple ways into different patterns of friendship (Ladd, 1983, 1988).

Social judgements

Friendship relations and social acceptance have a clear impact on social judgement and on interpretations of behavior, as revealed by laboratory investigations of simulated social conflicts. Children's social responses vary as a function of the quality of their relations. They respond differently to a peer's behavior, depending on how much they like or dislike the person who performs the act (Dodge, 1983). Children are likely to display more positive affect and prosocial behaviors when dealing with friends than with non-friends (Dodge, 1983; Masters & Furman, 1981). Juvonen (1991) reported that, when they stood them up, children expected their liked peers to be less angry at them and more forgiving than disliked classmates. The children believed that liked peers would be more understanding and considerate, but they also felt guilty when they broke a contact with friends, whereas no negative emotions were evoked in the same situation with a disliked peer (Juvonen, 1991). The emotions mediated between cognitions and behavior, and the expected emotional reaction (anger) was related to behavioral intentions attributed to self and others. Weiner and Handel (1985) found that children revealed or withheld the true reason for breaking a prior agreement, depending on the perceived likelihood of receiving an angry response from the other.

These trends can be explained, at least in part, by affective biases involved in causal reasoning (Juvonen, 1991). Several studies reported that when judging others' behavior, individuals tend to interpret liked persons' intentions more favorably than disliked persons' (Hymel, 1986; Waas & Honer, 1990). For example, Hymel found that children perceived unpopular peers to be more responsible for negative behaviors than liked peers. Children's beliefs that friendships are equal, cooperative, loyal, intimate, respectful, and reciprocal relations were shown to be likely to influence how they deal with friends and non-friends (Berndt, 1981; Furman & Bierman, 1984).

These results implied that feelings of loneliness may stem from different sources which, in combination, may undermine children's feelings of well-being (Parker & Asher, in press). A contribution to loneliness may be made by a lack of friends, or by friendships that fail to meet important relationship needs. Social judgement mediates experiences, further affecting and being affected by accompanying emotions.

Classroom climate, friendship, and loneliness

Research on peer relations has highlighted the role of same-age children as major contributors to the attributes of companionship networks and rejection relations. The systemic approach extended this perspective through focusing interest on characteristics of the learning environment -- the context where the examined peer relations are developed. It is well accepted that learning environments such as classes and schools affect not only the students' learning performance, but also have a clear impact on children's social rejections, cooperation, and relations in general. The systemic framework considers physical, cognitive, emotional, and social aspects of the learning milieu and their determinants and effects on the students' and teachers' functioning (Moos, 1987). Classroom climate affects the system members -- teachers and students -- in parallel ways. The teacher in particular, as a leader in this environment, often emphasizes and deemphasizes behaviors and expectations that have a clear contribution to the classroom climate. For example, substantial achievement gains in academic areas may occur in classes that accentuate learning performance and competition. However, educational systems that are lower in interpersonal warmth and student-teacher support and higher on control and strict disciplinary activities may promote tension, dissatisfaction, and absenteeism (Moos, 1987).

Similar results to those that were already described in the family climate discussion (see Chapter 3) were noted in the examination of the classroom climate, yielding the following three systemic dimensions:

Relationship: the relations between the classroom members -- how close, supportive or conflictual they are.

Personal growth: the aspects of individual growth emphasized within the class, enhancing competition between students, independence, and promoting cultural and intellectual involvement.

System maintenance: the rules and work habits within the classroom.

All these dimensions were linked to students' learning, functioning, and social relations. Teachers' impact on students' behavior within the school climate (Burke & McDonnell, 1992) was mediated through the attention given by teachers to order and organization (system-maintenance domain), their caring for students (relationship domain), and their emphasis on learning and academic achievements through curriculum development and implementation, design of instructional strategies, and material selection (personal growth domain). Yet, teachers at the same time are constantly affected by the students' functioning and behavior. Teachers' leadership has not only been closely linked to the teacher's own educational history, personality characteristics, and beliefs, but also can be seen as reflecting the continuous interactions with the students' characteristics within a reciprocal paradigm.

Teaching style

Role definitions of teachers have been related to various aspects of promoting knowledge and teaching new skills. The unique difficulties of students with disabilities make this role more critical and complicated, pinpointing educators' beliefs and attitudes related to disabilities, in addition to their needs for specific skills, training, and knowledge in order to be able to significantly address the difficulties of these students. The formulation of a teaching style and decisions regarding the focus of classroom activities are related to many aspects of teachers' own definitions of their role and performance. The adoption of a comprehensive approach to all aspects of student functioning that promote growth and adjustment, rather than the inclusion only of activities focused on learning and the acquirement of knowledge, can be instrumental in creating a classroom system conducive to students' well-being rather than to their loneliness and alienation.

In the classrooms, teachers structure academic lessons differently, allowing students to work either competitively, individually, or cooperatively. An understanding of these different climate styles may have a profound significance for identifying their impact on children at risk for social distress and loneliness.

Competitive climate. Students in a competitive classroom climate may feel themselves to be in a constant race to outperform others, and they may experience despair if they do not believe they have a chance of succeeding in the ongoing contest. The focus here is on students' personal achievement relative to other classmates, thus students' status reflects academic achievements and failures. The interrelations between students in such a classroom climate are centered around constant comparisons and competitiveness.

Individualistic climate. The emphasis of the individualistic approach to learning is on the presentation and evaluation of task achievement and individual goals, without continuous comparisons between students' achievements. Students seek outcomes that are personally beneficial and are encouraged to treat the goals and achievements of their classmates as irrelevant. However, in this setting, there is less reinforcement given to peer interactions and companionship. Students are encouraged to develop independent learning skills such as ignoring one another, working alone, and focusing only on their own work, in order to benefit from the solitary experience.

Cooperative climate. In the cooperative learning atmosphere, teachers structure tasks so that students will work together to accomplish shared goals. Students are assigned to small groups and instructed to work together. The learning goals can be reached only through the joint performance of peers (Johnson & Johnson, 1986). In this classroom climate, the learning efforts will be directed not only toward increasing one's knowledge-base, but also toward developing effective procedures for cooperative performance and learning in groups.

Different teaching methods have the potential to be related to students' feelings of loneliness. The disabled children within competitive environments may be expected to hold a reputation for having lower achievements and for being less respected and more rejected. Within a cooperative learning climate, some groups may reject disabled children who might interfere with the success of the joined task performance or affect its pace. The individualistic approach may enable students to achieve personal goals according to their own individual rate and may also increase children's capacity to be alone. However, in an individualistic climate, peer relations are not reinforced and supported. The teacher's role within each climate is critical for children with disabilities, to ensure the social experience and the support needed to develop a positive self-concept and satisfying social relations.

Loneliness and teacher attitudes

Research (Page, 1991a) has attempted to assess elementary school teachers' perceptions regarding students' loneliness. It was found that most teachers considered loneliness and social alienation to be a most important area in need of teacher intervention. In classrooms for students with learning disabilities (Unger, 1993), as can be seen on Figure 4.1, teachers viewed children's loneliness as more severe than that described by mothers or reported by the students themselves. It is not clear whether these teachers' perceptions represent a valid evaluation of the students' social reality, based on their day-to-day observations in class and compared to nondisabled students; or whether they reflect teachers' worries and concerns. Teachers expressed the feeling that they had not been adequately trained or prepared to deal with students' loneliness or social distress, and yet they assessed the problem as an extremely difficult one in need of highly professional skills (Page, 1991a). These perceptions among teachers may explain their reported sense of helplessness when discussing loneliness and their reluctance to become involved in treating children's social behavior and adjustment. Teachers expressed much concern over their lack of training in how to plan classroom climates to promote social relations, companionship, and students' social growth (Page, 1991a).

Discussions with teachers of disabled and nondisabled children held at Tel Aviv University revealed an additional source of teacher reluctance to deal with their students' loneliness experiences. Teachers talked about the children's social distress as reminding them of their own social difficulties in childhood. Those teachers who presented themselves as lonely persons felt both attracted and threatened by the need to be responsible for social change in the classroom. They expressed interest and even sympathy yet profound hesitation to become involved in a subject that they considered to be more clinically oriented than most academic subjects.

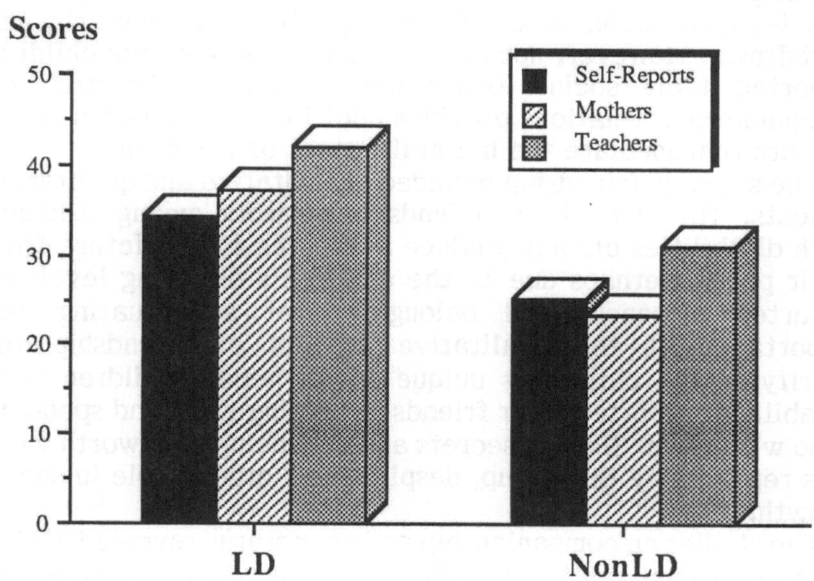

Figure 4.1 Loneliness scores according to self-reports and mother and teacher ratings

The holistic system-oriented framework can begin to capture the complexity of the socio-educational process in the classroom. This view suggests that the meaning and the outcome of educational systems must be considered in a broad social context (Walberg & Tsai, 1983), relating school and home environments as two interacting systems. It appears that the awareness and skills of the significant adults in the students' lives must be a central target for development in order to treat the special social needs of students with disabilities.

Conclusions

Social status and children's friendships were presented in this chapter as important predictors of the loneliness experience, in view of the consistent ratings of children with disabilities as less accepted by peers. The studies of peer status pinpointed the existence of five status groups of children: popular, rejected, neglected, controversial, and average. Many of the children with disabilities fall into the rejected and neglected status groups, with the rejected demonstrating more aggressive and disruptive behaviors, and the neglected being more shy and withdrawn. However, not all rejected and low-status children reported their social experience as lonely. Research on companionship relations provides additional information about factors that mediate the harmful impact of rejection.

The study of friendship included quantitative and qualitative aspects. The size of the friendship network among students with disabilities did not produce a differentiated picture from their peers, perhaps due to the children's differing levels of reported closeness and belonging, yet accentuating the importance of the qualitative aspects of friendship for clarifying the children's unique social needs. Children with disabilities reported their friends as helping them and spending time with them. Sharing secrets and enhancing self-worth were less reported by this group, despite their crucial role in social growth.

The studies on companionship and peer status revealed a wide range of social relations, reflecting personal differences and contextual conditions such as classroom climates, with different connections between peer relations, teacher-student interactions, and the loneliness experience. Attempts to further clarify individual differences call for exploration of subgroups among children with disabilities. Loneliness is experienced by withdrawn children as well as by aggressive ones. Predictors and characteristics within the different groups may pinpoint their specific needs and developmental paths.

Section III
A Subtyping Approach

5 Subtyping Approach to Loneliness Research

Social acceptance and the experience of loneliness have been considered negatively interrelated. Children who are more rejected by peers can be expected to feel more lonely. However, a comprehensive survey (Asher, Parkhurst, Hymel, & Williams, 1990) examining the relations between non-handicapped children's subjective experience of loneliness and their peer acceptance levels revealed only moderate (negative) correlations between peer acceptance and loneliness. This survey also focused attention on the wide variability of loneliness levels expressed by those children who were rejected by their peers. Many of the rejected children felt very lonely and dissatisfied with their social relations, yet others did not report a greater extent of loneliness experience when compared to their nonrejected peers.

Similar research results were reported in studies that examined the loneliness feelings of different special education groups such as students with learning disabilities (Margalit & Ben-Dov, 1992; Zehavi, 1992), mild mental retardation (Avrahami, 1992; Margalit & Ronen, 1993), and behavior disorders (Margalit, 1993a). These studies substantiated the inconsistent picture that emerged; not all disabled and nondisabled children who were poorly accepted by their peers found their social world to be lonely and dissatisfying. These two findings -- the extensive variability in loneliness scores and the moderate correlation between peer acceptance and loneliness -- supported the need to identify behavioral subtypes within the studied groups that differed in their degree of reported loneliness.

The problem of heterogeneity within the mild disabilities field has been widely acknowledged, leading to repeated attempts to organize the differing children into meaningful subgroups (Hooper & Willis, 1989; Kavale & Forness, 1992; Seigel & Metsala, 1992). Stone and LaGreca (1990), in their study of the social status difficulties among learning disabled students, stated that the vast research evidence already existing in this area calls for a move from general comparisons of disabled and nondisabled populations to a more fine-grain analysis of subgroups within the studied population. This approach may promise not only a greater theoretical understanding of the children's dysfunctions, but may also be a valuable guide in the search for more individualized intervention programming that attends to unique needs and abilities.

In this chapter, research will be presented within an attempt to differentiate and identify distinct subgroups of lonely and non-lonely children within different groups of disabled children. This proposed subtyping model consists of an extension and adaptation of two existing models for subtyping children: (a) the subtyping model for aggressive children (Dodge & Coie, 1987; Landau & Milich, 1985; Ledingham, 1981; Margalit, 1988); and (b) the subtyping model for rejected children (Parkhurst & Asher, 1992; Rubin, LeMare, & Lollis, 1990; Taylor, Asher, & Williams, 1987).

Following the description of the two existing models, two studies will be presented. The first study identified subgroups among learning disabled children, and the second study compared subgroups among two samples of male students: those with behavior difficulties and those with learning disabilities.

Subtyping aggressive children

Physical and verbal expressions of aggression, non-compliance, destructiveness, and negative relations with peers and/or adults comprise the well-accepted definition of behavior disorders. These characteristics were reported by studies of normal and clinical populations in different countries, across the span of childhood from preschool age through adolescence (Achenbach, 1982; Margalit, 1988; Quay, 1983). Persistence of aggressive behavior for boys and girls over time has been established through longitudinal studies (Cairns & Cairns, 1984; Kazdin, 1987; Prage, Greenbaum, Silver, & Friedman, 1992). Hard-to-manage preschoolers with conduct problems were defined as a group at high risk for clinically significant problems in later childhood (Eyberg, 1992). Aggressive behaviors violate major social rules and expectations within the child's social systems (such as the family and the school) and often also reflect actions against these environments, including both persons and property (Kazdin, 1987). Ineffective parenting and poor peer relations elicited by the children's aggressive behaviors may contribute to the maintenance of the disruptive behavior over time (Vuchinich, Bank, & Patterson, 1992).

Research on relations between social status and disruptive behavior has revealed inconsistent patterns, with some studies reporting peer rejection and lower social status for students with aggressive behavior, and others not (Landau & Milich, 1985). Several attempts to identify unique subgroups of aggressive children have been reported.

Aggressive/withdrawn versus "pure" aggressive subgroups

Within an approach positing the heterogeneous nature of this group of children, Ledingham (1981) distinguished between two subgroups of aggressive youngsters. The first subgroup was viewed as "pure" aggressive children -- those who did not reveal additional attention difficulties. The second subgroup was labeled aggressive/withdrawn children -- those demonstrating higher levels of distractibility and problems in sustaining attention and completing tasks. Milich and Landau's (1984) findings, that the social status of purely aggressive children was higher than that of the aggressive/withdrawn ones, supported Ledingham's subtyping conceptualization. The purely aggressive group was observed as engaged in both positive and negative social interactions and as spending less time in solitary play. The aggressive/withdrawn group was less liked by peers, spent more time in solitary play, and also evidenced more hyperactive behavior, similarly to Loney and Milich's (1982) descriptions of a hyperactive/aggressive subgroup.

Several studies (Dodge & Coie, 1987; Landau & Milich, 1985; Ledingham & Schwartzman, 1984; Milich & Landau, 1984) have corroborated this subgrouping, identifying the subset of purely aggressive children as having a controversial sociometric status -- rated both as accepted and as rejected by peers -- and as having at least an average level of leadership and problem-solving skills. The subset of children with aggressive/withdrawn behavior was identified as sociometrically rejected and as evidencing attributional biases as well as social-cognitive and problem-solving deficits (see Chapter 2).

Introverted aggressive versus extroverted aggressive subgroups

A similar approach for subtyping aggressive children was presented in Margalit's (1988) study, within Eysenck and Eysenck's (1985) model of individual personality differences and Achenbach's (1982) conceptualization of child psychopathology. Margalit's investigation of students who exhibited aggressive behavior pointed out the existence of two distinct subgroups: introverted and extroverted. The introverted aggressive subgroup of children, analogous to the aforementioned withdrawn/aggressive subgroup, demonstrated more hyperactive behavior, greater dependence on others, lower maturity, and less consideration. Lower academic achievements and social status were also reported for this subgroup in comparison to the extroverted subgroup. The extroverted aggressive subgroup of children, analogous to the aforementioned purely aggressive subgroup, demonstrated hostility levels similar to those of the introverted subgroup, yet the extroverted children revealed more interpersonal understanding and self-control and were viewed by their peers as more popular.

Attribution processes in aggressive subgrouping

Attribution research on aggressive children provided additional validation to the differentiation between the two groups of aggressive children: the aggressive-rejected subgroup and the aggressive-non-rejected subgroup. The ways these children provide causal interpretations to events further clarify the cognitive model of reciprocal aggressive behavior (Bierman, 1986a, 1986b; Dodge, 1986) postulating that aggressive children acquire an expectation that peers will behave toward them in hostile ways. This expectation causes them to respond quickly and to attend selectively to hostile cues, thus overattributing hostility to peers' behaviors toward them. Their biased attributions cause them to respond aggressively, which in turn leads to retaliatory aggression from peers, confirming the original expectations.

Research has revealed a unique processing difficulty evidenced by children in the aggressive-rejected subgroup (Keltikangas-Jarvinen & Kangas, 1988). These children were noted for their difficulty in detecting constructive alternatives to aggressive behavior. Aggressive-rejected children expressed more hostile attributions and fewer positive attributions than did aggressive children who were not rejected, and were also found to engage in fewer positive behaviors with peers than did aggressive non-rejected children (Gottman, Gonso, & Rasmussen, 1975).

Studies on positive social behaviors added another perspective to the understanding of the development of attribution processing. Children who evidenced a higher level of positive social behavior (such as cooperating, sharing, and joining in) were more likely to express positive attributions and to receive more positive behavioral responses and acceptance ratings from their peers (Coie, 1985; Coie & Kupersmidt, 1983; Masters & Furman, 1981). Similarly to negative social attributions that enter into the cycle of aggression and retaliation, deficits in prosocial behaviors may also lead to distortions in interpretations and to fewer opportunities for positive peer attributions of interactions. Peer-accepted children who are rated as having better social-cognitive skills and who display more prosocial behaviors may be viewed as participating in a positive socialization cycle, where their positive behaviors cause peers to further react positively to them. Aggressive-rejected children do not participate to the same degree in this positive socialization cycle. Differences between the rejected and the nonrejected children's interpretations of their peers' positive behaviors may account in part for the differences in the behavior of the two subgroups of aggressive children.

Hughes, Robinson, and Moore's (1991) research further clarified the uniqueness in attribution style of the aggressive-rejected subgroup. Their study reflected the value of considering the extent of the child's involvement within the examined conditions. In this study, the children were presented with two situations that differed regarding the degree to which the child was personally involved. The first situation consisted of the presentation of a hypothetical story of children's interrelations (i.e., under a condition of low personal involvement), where the child's responses reflected his or her ability to discriminate others' intentions in social situations involving positive outcomes. The second situation, where the child received an unexpected gift (i.e., under a condition of high personal involvement), can be viewed as similar to a real-life situation. In the latter situation, aggressive-rejected children exhibited a significant tendency to underattribute positive intent to peers' behavior, whereas this tendency was not significant in the hypothetical situation. Thus, in a real-life situation in which peers' actions directly affected them, aggressive-rejected children responded in accordance with their personal belief that others act with less positive intentions toward them.

Self-esteem of aggressive groups

The comparison of three subgroups of children -- aggressive, withdrawn, and aggressive/withdrawn -- revealed that children who were solely aggressive had higher self-esteem scores and more popularity than did the other two subgroups (Landau & Milich, 1985; Ledingham, 1981; Schneider & Leitenberg, 1989). One possible explanation for this finding is that self-esteem has been associated with peer status, and aggressive children were more popular than aggressive/withdrawn children. Unpopularity and low self-esteem most likely help to reinforce one another. Another possible explanation presented by Schneider and Leitenberg (1989) for the higher self-esteem of aggressive children was related to their more self-enhancing attributional response style. The aggressive subgroup had a greater tendency to attribute their hypothetical successful experience to their own personal ability, reflecting higher self-esteem and lower depressive tendencies (Schneider & Leitenberg, 1989). The different patterns of aggressive behaviors may be conceptualized as alternative developmental pathways, where the withdrawn/aggressive behaviors lead to later loneliness and social rejection (Rubin, LeMare, & Lollis, 1990).

Reactive versus proactive grouping

Another approach to subtyping aggressive behavior focused interest on the two types of differential origins for manifestations of aggression and hostility (Dodge & Coie, 1987): proactive aggression and reactive aggression:

Proactive (instrumental) aggression is deliberate, controlled, goal-directed behavior such as a display of power to achieve an external goal. Behaviors such as dominance and bullying, typifying this type of aggression, seem to occur without immediate provocation. Proactive aggression is considered to be an effective instrument for achieving specific outcomes related to internal goals.

Reactive aggression is a less controlled outburst of angry behavior that appears to be a defensive reaction to frustration or rejection. This second type involves an aggressive expression of hostility, as often prompted by the child's interpretation that another individual has provoked him or her and has hostile intent. Thus, reactive aggressive behavior may be viewed as a defensive response to a perceived threatening stimulus, with the function of relieving the perceived threat rather than of achieving some internal goal. Within the social-information processing model of social competence, some types of inefficient and inaccurate processing will lead the child to retaliate aggressively in response to conflicts and provocations by peers. Dodge and Coie's (1987) study suggested that children who have a tendency to make inaccurate interpretations due to their processing deficits are likely to display high levels of reactive aggression. Reactive aggression appeared to be the distinguishing factor for the presence or absence of social skill problems (Day, Bream, & Pal, 1992), and teachers viewed these children as unable to control their aggressive impulses and as less liked by adults and peers.

The different treatment needs suggested for these two groups further illuminate their differentiation. It appears that reactive children are seen as having more social skills deficits and as in need of social skills training concentrating on metacognitive self-evaluation and self-training. The proactive group was considered to need treatments promoting the development of alternate behaviors for achieving desired outcomes and of the internalization of values other than aggression (Day, Bream, & Pal, 1992).

In conclusion, different forms of aggressive behavior appear to originate from different cognitive processes. In line with the information processing view of social behavior (Dodge, 1986; Hughes, Robinson, & Moore, 1991), children's cognitive processing of social cues in a situation determines in part their response. The differentiated subtyping of aggressive children may clarify the distinct patterns of processing difficulties and behavior patterns among the various subgroups of children who evidence aggressive behavior. Differences in personality style and unique social cognition patterns were found to be related to individual differences in the quality of interpersonal relations among children (Dodge & Coie, 1987). These differences were also expressed in the children's loneliness reports. The withdrawn aggressive children were lonely, whereas the purely aggressive children were well accepted by their peers and did not report loneliness.

Subtyping rejected children

The heterogeneity of rejected children also calls for the development of a subtyping model. Data on social acceptance and rejection provided by behavioral observations and sociometric assessments have revealed that two subgroups can be identified: (a) an active, aggressive, disruptive subgroup, and (b) a passive, submissive, lonely, and withdrawn subgroup (Cantrell & Prinz, 1985; Coie & Kupersmidt, 1983; Dodge, 1983; Dodge, Coie, & Brakke, 1982; Parkhurst & Asher, 1992). Submissive, socially rejected children showed higher levels of loneliness and worries about humiliation and rejection and were not high on either aggressiveness or disruptiveness. The aggressive-rejected students showed high levels of disruptiveness but less submissiveness or shyness, and they felt relatively less lonely (Parkhurst & Asher, 1992).

This identification of subgroups was found consistent over different age levels and was also identified for a sample of students with educable mental retardation (Taylor, Asher, & Williams, 1987). The results revealed that, although the educable mentally retarded sample as a group was generally dissatisfied with their social interrelations, the submissive subgroup reported much more social dissatisfaction.

In line with the externalizing versus internalizing patterns of child psychopathology (Achenbach, 1982; Hymel, Rubin, Rowden, & LeMare, 1990), two distinct subgroups of socially rejected nondisabled children were identified (Rubin, LeMare,& Lollis, 1990). The first subgroup of rejected children, rated by significant adults as demonstrating internalizing problems, consisted of children characterized as anxious, apprehensive, timid, isolated, extremely lacking in social assertiveness, and socially withdrawn. The second subgroup of rejected children, rated by adults as evidencing externalizing problems, was composed of aggressive, hostile, and disruptive children.

Another study supported the consistency of these trends, providing a description of two subgroups of socially rejected children (Rubin & Mills, 1988). The first type consisted of passive, anxious, isolated students, with social anxiety and negative self-perceptions of competence, who are often rejected by peers and may be at risk for developing loneliness. The second type consisted of active, immature children whose teachers viewed them as impulsive and aggressive (Rubin & Clark, 1983) and who were also found to be disliked and rejected by peers (Rubin & Daniels-Beirness, 1983).

It can be concluded that the subtyping models of aggressive children and of rejected children seem complementary, consistently leading to the identification of three subgroups: two subgroups of externalizing, disruptive children (a purely aggressive, non-lonely subgroup, whose social status was found controversial; and a rejected, lonely, aggressive subgroup) and one internalizing subgroup (withdrawn, rejected, lonely children).

Subtyping of students with learning disabilities

Students with learning disabilities have often been recognized as having social deficits and needing social skills training, yet little research has focused on how they feel about their social interrelations. A recent study (Margalit & Al-Yagon, in press) has attempted to relate maladjustment subgroupings with subjective loneliness experiences and measures of social relations.

It should be remembered that learning disability research has highlighted not only these students' academic problems, but also their major psychosocial difficulties of a heterogenous nature. These children were often found as demonstrating social skill deficiencies, maladjusted behavior, and low peer acceptance. At the same time, research has also demonstrated that a significant number of students with learning disabilities appear to be psychosocially indistinguishable from their nondisabled peers (Bryan, Pearl, & Fallon, 1989; Pearl, 1992). These inconsistent empirical findings, implying the possible existence of a learning disability subgroup evidencing appropriate skills within the psychosocial domain, emphasizes the value of identifying social-emotional subtypes among these students, using social and behavioral maladjustment variables as the criteria for subtyping. When heterogeneous groups of students with learning disabilities were subtyped, different social profiles emerged (Hooper & Willis, 1989), emphasizing conduct disorders as the most salient social adjustment problem experienced by these students (Epstein, Bursuck, & Cullinan, 1985; Hooper & Willis, 1989).

In line with the two subgrouping models for aggression and rejection (Landau & Milich, 1985; Parkhurst & Asher, 1992; Rubin, LeMare, & Lollis, 1990), Margalit and Al-Yagon's (in press) study identified patterns of social-emotional subgroups among students with learning disabilities, regarding their internalizing/externalizing behavior difficulties and feelings of loneliness. Four subgroups were identified in this study of 122 learning disabled children, with ages ranging from 9.0 to 15.0 years (M = 12.50, SD = 1.53). The groups included two subgroups of non-lonely students -- those with externalizing tendencies and those who were relatively adjusted -- and two subgroups of lonely students -- those with externalizing maladjustment tendencies and those with internalizing maladjustment tendencies. Their social skills, peer ratings, and number of friends were also examined and compared. Figure 5.1 presents the comparison of loneliness and maladjustment measures between the four different subgroups of children with learning disabilities.

Subgroup A: Non-lonely/externalizing

The first subgroup of learning disabled children included 17 students, 13 males and 4 females, consisting of 13.9% of the sample (ages: M = 12.59, SD = 1.23). This small group of students demonstrated high levels of externalizing maladjustment but felt socially competent, with the lowest levels of internalizing maladjustment, and seldom experiencing loneliness.

They had good social skills and felt they had many friends with whom to share their time. These students were in fact well accepted by their peers and were regarded by their teachers as often initiating social interactions. Yet the teachers reported this subgroup to be low in cooperation with children and adults and in self-control.

Subgroup B: Non-lonely/internalizing

The second subgroup included 32 students, 20 males and 12 females, consisting of 26.2% of the sample (ages: $M = 11.97$, $SD = 1.61$). More than one quarter of the sample may be viewed as a group of students whose major problems focused on academic areas, while its social-emotional status can be regarded as relatively age-appropriate. Its members viewed themselves as socially skilled and low in loneliness. Teachers rated them as cooperative in their interrelations and low in externalizing maladjustment, and peers viewed them as socially accepted.

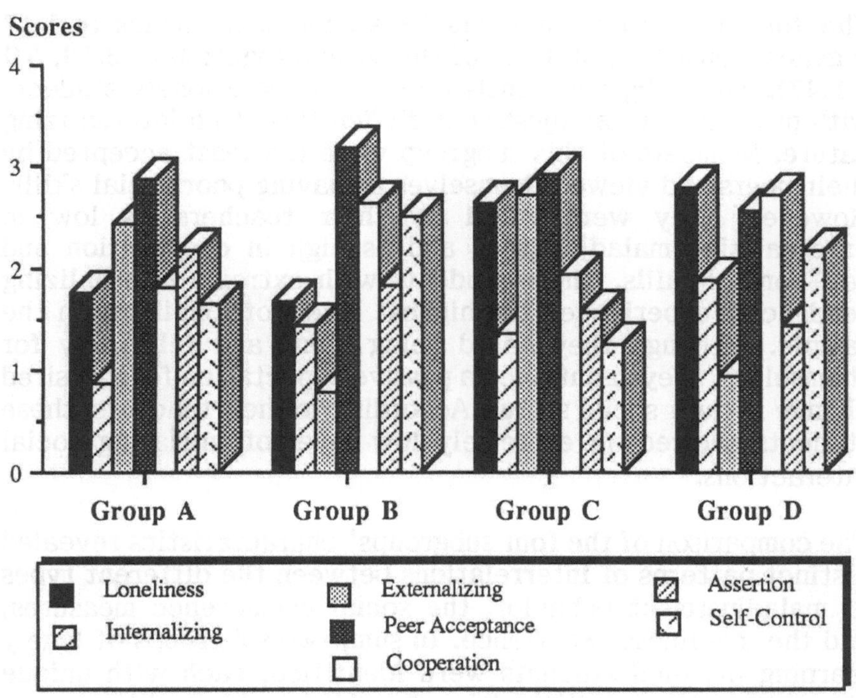

Figure 5.1 Comparison of loneliness, social competence, and maladjustment measures between four subgroups of children with learning disabilities

Subgroup C: Lonely/highly externalizing

The third subgroup was comprised of 35 students, 28 males and 7 females, consisting of 28.7% of the sample (ages: $M = 12.18$, $SD = 1.40$). These students perceived themselves as lonely individuals, and their teachers rated them as demonstrating extremely maladjusted externalizing behavior and the lowest levels of self-control skills. They were not accepted by their peers and reported their loneliness and social dissatisfaction. The students in this subgroup were aware of their social difficulties and wished to acquire more friends. They also viewed themselves as less socially skilled, often failing to control their frustrations and anger, and easily getting into trouble.

Subgroup D: Highly lonely/highly internalizing

The fourth subgroup included 38 students, 21 males and 17 females, consisting of 31.2% of the sample (ages: $M = 13.18$, $SD = 1.47$). This subgroup consisted of extremely lonely students with pronounced maladjustment difficulties of an internalizing nature. Members of this subgroup were the least accepted by their peers and viewed themselves as having poor social skills. However, they were rated by their teachers as low in externalizing maladjustment and as high in cooperation and self-control skills. These students with extreme internalizing tendencies experienced the highest levels of loneliness in the sample. Although they hated being alone and felt sorry for themselves, they maintained a passive expectation for a desired change in their social status. According to their teachers, these students showed an extremely low level of initiating social interactions.

The comparison of the four subgroups' characteristics revealed distinct patterns of interrelations between the different types of maladjustment behavior, the social competence measures, and the loneliness experience. In sum, two subgroups of lonely learning disabled students were identified, each with unique characteristics and difficulties. In addition, it should be noted that even within the subgroup of relatively socially adjusted children with learning disabilities, some amount of loneliness was expressed.

Subtyping comparisons for groups with learning disabilities and behavior disorders

In line with McKinney's (1988) recommendation to explore the adaptive and maladaptive behavior of children with mild disabilities in comparison to that of other diagnostic groups, the four-group classification model was used to explore the differentiation between students who have learning disabilities and students with behavior disorders (Margalit, 1993a). Earlier research on the differentiation between these two groups of students regarding behavioral, cognitive, and academic functioning has resulted in inconsistent conclusions (Fessler, Rosenberg, & Rosenberg, 1991; Margalit, 1992; Sabornie, Kauffman, Ellis, Marshall, & Elksnin, 1987-8; Sabornie & Thomas, 1989). In Margalit's (1993b) study, the subtyping model was examined with regard to various measures of social adaptation. The sample consisted of 170 male students, divided into two groups:

1. *Students with learning disabilities*: 81 boys from ten special education classes for students with learning disabilities, with ages ranging from 10.0 to 15.0 years (M = 12.32, SD = 1.43).

2. *Students with behavior disorders*: 89 boys from ten special education classes for students with behavior disorders, with ages ranging from 9.6 to 15.0 years (M = 12.49, SD = 1.80).

The two groups did not differ in their loneliness or peer acceptance levels. However the comparisons between the learning disabled and behavior disordered groups revealed that the latter group demonstrated more extreme scores on both types of maladjustment: Students with behavior disorders were found to be more extreme in their internalizing behavior and in their externalizing behavior. In addition, they rated themselves as having better social skills than did students with learning disabilities. Teachers rated students with behavior disorders as having lower levels of self-control.

The subtyping procedure for both samples together in Margalit's (1993b) study was identical to that used in the aforementioned subtyping research for a learning disabled sample alone (Margalit & Al-Yagon, in press). In the comparative study, teachers' ratings of externalizing and internalizing maladjustment and students' feelings of loneliness were used to identify subgroups for the two samples together as one group, through a K-means clustering analysis procedure on the basis of their similarity over the teacher-rated (externalizing and internalizing) maladjustment measures and the student-reported loneliness scores. Four subgroups of students were identified. Case studies for each subgroup were added to exemplify the usefulness of the subtyping procedure, using data from children's and teachers' questionnaires and interviews.

Subgroup A: Non-lonely/externalizing

The first subgroup included 12 students with learning disabilities, consisting of 14.8% of the learning disabled sample (ages: M = 12.33, SD = 1.30) and 27 students with behavior disorders, consisting of 30.3% of the behavior disordered sample (ages: M = 12.56, SD = 1.81). This subgroup of students reported lower levels of loneliness feelings and demonstrated high levels of externalizing difficulties and a moderate level of internalizing maladjustment. The students felt socially competent, initiated social interactions, and experienced lower levels of loneliness. They were accepted by peers and felt they had many friends. However, they were regarded by their teachers as not cooperative and less controlled.

Case studies for subgroup A

> *Noam was a 9-year-old boy with severe behavior disorders in the fourth grade. His main difficulty was his uncontrolled aggressive behavior. He often expressed dissatisfaction, became angry easily, and reached a state of uncontrolled tantrums very quickly. Children attempted to avoid disagreeing with him, knowing that he often threatened, pushed, and cursed them. His academic achievements were as expected for his age level.*
>
> *His social status was considered controversial. He was accepted by many of his classmates but was also rejected by many of them. He considered a friend to be "a good boy who helps me in everything, and we can play together." He also understood the meaning of loneliness -- staying alone and feeling sad. He said that a lonely child can be*

identified by "looking at his face, and by seeing how he stands." Yet, he could not imagine a situation in which a child could be with other children but feel lonely. It is not clear if his limited understanding of the loneliness concept reflected a simplistic and less mature conceptualization or defensive tendencies.

He did not consider himself to be a lonely child. As another expression of defensive tendencies, he could not remember even once feeling lonely. He stated that he always felt an integral part of the group and was certain that he could always find somebody with whom to play. He considered companionship to be a very important factor in his life, and he was ready when needed to search actively for company, even of young children.

Ram was a 10-year-old boy with learning disabilities, in the fifth grade, whose main problems centered around his constant anger and hostile behavior. He was viewed by his teacher as often demonstrating verbal and physical aggression toward adults and peers. He became angry easily, often arguing, fighting, and losing his temper. Ram considered himself as socially competent, as usually "getting along" with peers, and as having many friends. The sociometric scores validated his social perceptions, revealing that he was highly accepted by peers. Several students in school were considered to be his "best" friends because they "hang around together all the time -- laughing, playing, and doing everything together." Both his questionnaire ratings and interview data indicated that Ram did not feel lonely. He did not deny its possibility: "It can happen, but not often." Ram understood the meaning of loneliness, saying that the experience of loneliness seemed to be possible even when in a group "when nobody pays attention to you or talks to you." When he felt alone, Ram spent time in various solitary activities such as watching television, playing with his computer, or even trying to fall asleep. When asked how he would advise a child who does not have friends, Ram emphatically stated that the child should try to avoid doing "bad things like hitting, cursing, and making faces," detailing a number of aggressive behaviors that the teacher had described in relation to his own behavior difficulties.

The cases of Noam and Ram were derived from the aggressive, externalizing subgroup of students. Similar patterns of social interrelations emerged from the descriptions, regardless of the fact that Noam had only behavioral and disciplinary difficulties and was identified as a student with behavior disorders, whereas Ram was identified as a learning disabled student whose oral reading mastery was slow and whose reading comprehension was significantly lower than expected for his age level. However, Ram's major difficulties were also centered around his disruptive behavior. The group comparisons between students with learning disabilities and students with behavior disorders revealed relatively higher levels of loneliness among the students of the first subgroup. The perceptions of loneliness among the students with behavior disorders were extremely low. Several children even insisted that they never felt lonely.

Subgroup B: Non-lonely/internalizing

The second subgroup included 21 students with learning disabilities, consisting of 25.9% of the learning disabled sample (ages: M = 11.67, SD = 1.32) and 16 students with behavior disorders, consisting of 18.0% of the behavior disordered sample (ages: M = 13.25, SD = 1.69). These students viewed themselves as low in loneliness and were rated by their teachers as low in externalizing maladjustment, with moderate internalizing maladjustment behavior. More than in any other subgroup, these students were accepted by their peers. Similarly to students in subgroup A, they viewed themselves and were rated by their teachers as having good social skills. No significant differences were found between the students with learning disabilities and with behavior disorders in this subgroup with regard to loneliness levels.

Case studies for subgroup B

> *Ilan was a 15-year-old tenth-grade student with behavior difficulties whose teacher viewed him as extremely cooperative, with social skills appropriate to his age group, although sometimes he appeared sad. Although in the first years of school he had expressed much anger and sadness, currently he was considered friendly and cooperative. Relative to the other children in his special*

class he seemed well-behaved, although the teacher still felt worried about the long periods that he seemed passive and anxious and needed much adult attention and encouragement to join the group. He never answered back to adults and seemed very sensitive to others' needs, but also vulnerable to others' insults. When hurt or teased, he sometimes even cried. He liked school, having four good friends with whom he often played. They lived not far from his home and often met in the afternoons. In class he felt liked by peers, and his sociometric rating validated his feelings. Sometimes he felt lonely, but not often. At such times, he reported that he would go home, take his skateboard, and play with it outside. The teacher viewed him as a relatively self-controlled student who initiated social relations with peers, and his behavior within his special class for children with behavior disorders was considered adaptive. Yet from time to time he still expressed anxiety and depressive moods. His learning achievements were poor, seeming to reflect years of emotional difficulties and introverted maladjustment.

Gal was a 14-year-old student with learning disabilities in the eighth grade whose teacher described him as liked by his peers and well-behaved in class, although he seemed restless at times. The sociometric assessment reflected that his peers accepted and liked him. He himself felt that he had many friends and mentioned six good friends. His self-reported social skills rating was also relatively high. Gal described a good friend as "somebody who helps you, plays with you, and stays together with you." During an interview, he said that he did not often feel lonely and that when he had lonely moments, usually at home, he felt mainly bored. When he felt lonely, he tried to cheer himself up (i.e., active coping with mood), watch television, or read (i.e., finding alternative solitary activities that may be satisfying). Gal recommended that other children should, in order to attain friends, "laugh a lot, go out a lot with friends, act happy, and try to do what they want you to do."

In sum, Ilan and Gal were students in a subgroup of introverted yet relatively well-adjusted students. Both had social skills appropriate to their age group, were accepted by their peers, appeared to understand the meaning of loneliness, and reported having developed effective means of coping.

Subgroup C: Lonely/highly externalizing

The third subgroup included 28 students with learning disabilities, consisting of 34.6% of the learning disabled sample (ages: M = 12.14, SD = 1.27) and 33 students with behavior disorders, consisting of 37.1% of the behavior disordered sample (ages: M = 12.24, SD = 1.86). These students perceived themselves as lonely individuals, and their teachers rated them as demonstrating extremely maladjusted externalizing behavior and moderately maladjusted internalizing behavior. This subgroup of lonely students was noted by its behavior difficulties. Teachers rated these students as demonstrating the lowest levels of self-control. They were less accepted by their peers and were aware of their social difficulties and wished to gain friendships, yet failed to control their frustration and anger, and easily became provoked and got into trouble. No significant differences were found in the level of loneliness in this subgroup, between the students with learning disabilities and with behavior disorders.

Case studies for subgroup C

Ofer was a 15-year-old male student with behavior disorders in the tenth grade who reported feeling very lonely, and his teacher viewed him as demonstrating externalizing behavior difficulties with a hyperactive and restless behavior style. Ofer's aggressive behavior toward peers and adults was often related to his impulsiveness and difficulty in delaying satisfaction or dealing with frustration. He seemed to request constant attention (positive and/or negative) from children and adults in class and at home, easily becoming angry, arguing, quarrelling, answering back to children and adults without any differentiation, and bullying peers. Ofer recognized his social difficulties, felt alienated within his peer group, and expressed his anger at being isolated. His sociometric scores were low, and the teacher also reported that he was rejected by peers.

On the loneliness questionnaire, Ofer's scores were very high. When he was asked to describe a friend, all he could say was "somebody who comes over to my house, and I go to his," reflecting a very narrow concept of friendship provision. He reported that most of his free time at home was spent lonely and watching TV. Although his companionship conceptualization was simplistic, wherein he considered just being with somebody as an answer to loneliness, he kept complaining that he was alone, bored, and isolated. He recognized the need to initiate social contacts and to invite children "to go with each other, to develop contact" but his words seemed meaningless to him -- merely words that he had learned but did not know how to apply, lacking sufficient skills or energy to initiate an attempt toward social interactions.

Ben was a 13-year-old boy with learning disabilities in the seventh grade whose teacher rated him as evidencing good cooperation skills with adults but low self-control and pronounced externalizing behavior difficulties. Ben was described as a student who became angry easily until the point of losing his temper, often quarrelling, arguing, and threatening others, especially peers. He rated himself as having strong feelings of loneliness and low social skills, demonstrating his awareness of his difficulty in controlling anger. He mentioned having only one good friend, a boy in the neighborhood. Ben expected a good friend to "help you when you need help, and also to be nice to you." He remembered times "when everybody seemed to have a good time but I ended up by myself." His advice in order to have friends was "to be nice, not to make trouble." When he was alone he reported either staying at home to watch television (i.e., a solitary alternative activity) or going out to visit friends (i.e., active coping).

Ofer and Ben were very lonely students with an externalizing aggressive behavior style, representing a more reactive than instrumental aggressive style. Ben expressed a wish to have friends and seemed ready to invest efforts in establishing social relations. Ofer seemed to be a more hyperactive, disruptive youngster who viewed his situation as hopeless. The similarity in levels of behavior difficulties between the learning disabled and behavior disordered children in this subgroup was notable, substantiating the value of the subtyping approach rather than an approach based on clinical groups.

Subgroup D: Highly lonely/highly internalizing

The fourth subgroup included 20 students with learning disabilities, consisting of 24.7% of the learning disabled sample (ages: M = 13.25, SD = 1.45) and 13 students with behavior disorders, consisting of 14.6% of the behavior disordered sample (ages: M = 12.08, SD = 1.71). The students in this subgroup felt most lonely and were rated by their teachers as demonstrating the highest levels of internalizing maladjustment, along with low scores on the externalizing measure. The students with behavior disorders in this subgroup felt the highest levels of loneliness, viewed themselves as socially incompetent, and were the least accepted by peers. Although they hated staying alone and felt sorry for themselves, they remained passive in their expectation for the desired change in their social status. Their teacher viewed them as more self-controlled and cooperative than in the subgroups with externalizing maladjustment, yet remarked on their extremely low social initiation.

Case studies for subgroup D

> *Eli was a 14-year-old boy with behavior disorders in the ninth grade who viewed himself as extremely lonely and was described by his teacher as isolated in the class. He felt helpless when asked how he could change his social situation, since he seldom initiated activities, never asked for help, and attempted to avoid social interrelations. He was rejected or ignored by peers and rarely seemed cooperative.*
>
> *Eli himself said that he hated school and that he knew for sure that nobody in class liked him. He said that he had nobody with whom to play or even to talk. He felt isolated and outside the "gang." He considered it very difficult to find new friends but also had no old friends. If he could, he preferred staying home, watching TV, and feeling sad. The only activity that he found interesting and worth being involved in was computer activities. He was always ready to spend hours with computer games, at home or school.*
>
> *The teacher knew through his psychological evaluation that Eli had good intellectual abilities, yet his academic achievements were very low due to his lack of motivation. For Eli, the meaning of a friend was "somebody who will help you do your homework." However, he did not seem*

very enthusiastic to have a friend. His cooperation during the interview was limited. He talked in short sentences, preferred avoiding direct questions, and needed constant encouragement to continue answering.

Raz was an 11-year-old learning disabled student in the fifth grade who felt very lonely and whose behavior difficulties were described by his teacher as mainly internalizing. His cooperation with adults was rated as high, and he almost never exhibited aggressive or hyperactive behavior at school. Yet his cooperation with peers was very limited, and he was rejected by them, rarely initiating social interactions. He himself rated his social skills as low and said that he never shared his feelings (either positive or negative) with his peers, nor did he ask for adult or peer assistance when in need. For Raz the meaning of a friend was "somebody who will help you when you need it." His longing for friends was expressed in his statement, "When you are with other children you cannot feel lonely." He admitted that he often felt lonely but did not try to do anything to change it. Whenever he felt lonely, Raz waited passively, hoping that "somehow, somebody will come play with me."

Eli and Raz were lonely, introverted, and passive students who were rejected by their classmates and who did not actively attempt to change their situation. They seemed to lack a repertoire of effective coping strategies to deal with their loneliness feelings. Within this subgroup the scores of loneliness were extremely high, and the comparison between students with learning disabilities and those with behavior disorders revealed that those in the latter group reported even more extreme levels of loneliness than did those in the former.

Group comparisons

Figure 5.2 presents the mean scores for the two clinical categories of children in the four subgroups, focusing attention on the loneliness and adjustment measures. In subgroup A the loneliness scores were low, and the scores for the children with behavior disorders were even lower. In subgroup D, the loneliness scores were extremely high, with those of the children with behavior disorders even higher than those of the children with learning disabilities. It seems that, although mean sample scores of loneliness did not differentiate between students with learning disabilities and those with behavior disorders, the four-group subtyping demonstrated the differences, with more extreme scores of the students with behavior disorders.

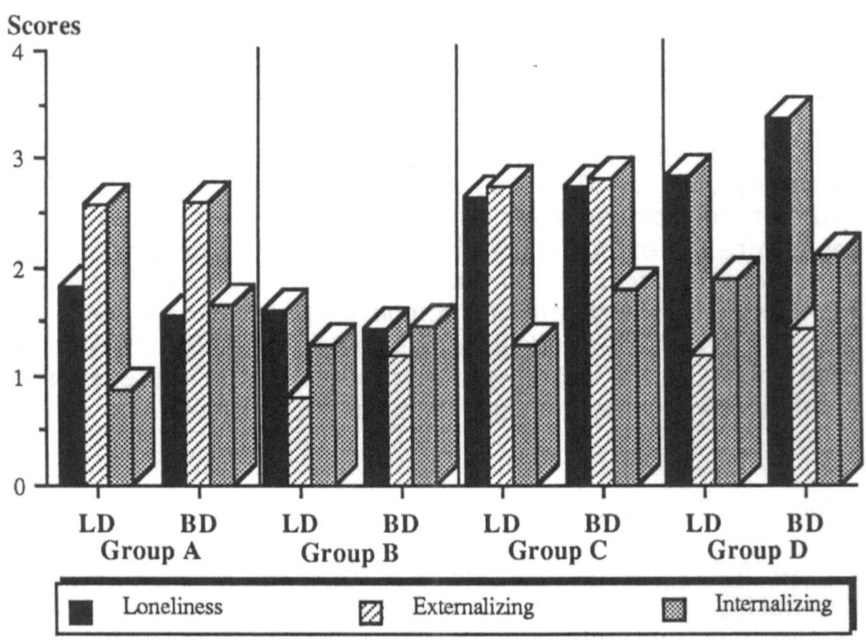

Figure 5.2 Mean scores for the children with learning disabilities and the children with behavior disorders in the four subgroups

Significant differences were also found in the proportions of the two clinical groups within the different subgroups, as can be seen on Figure 5.3.

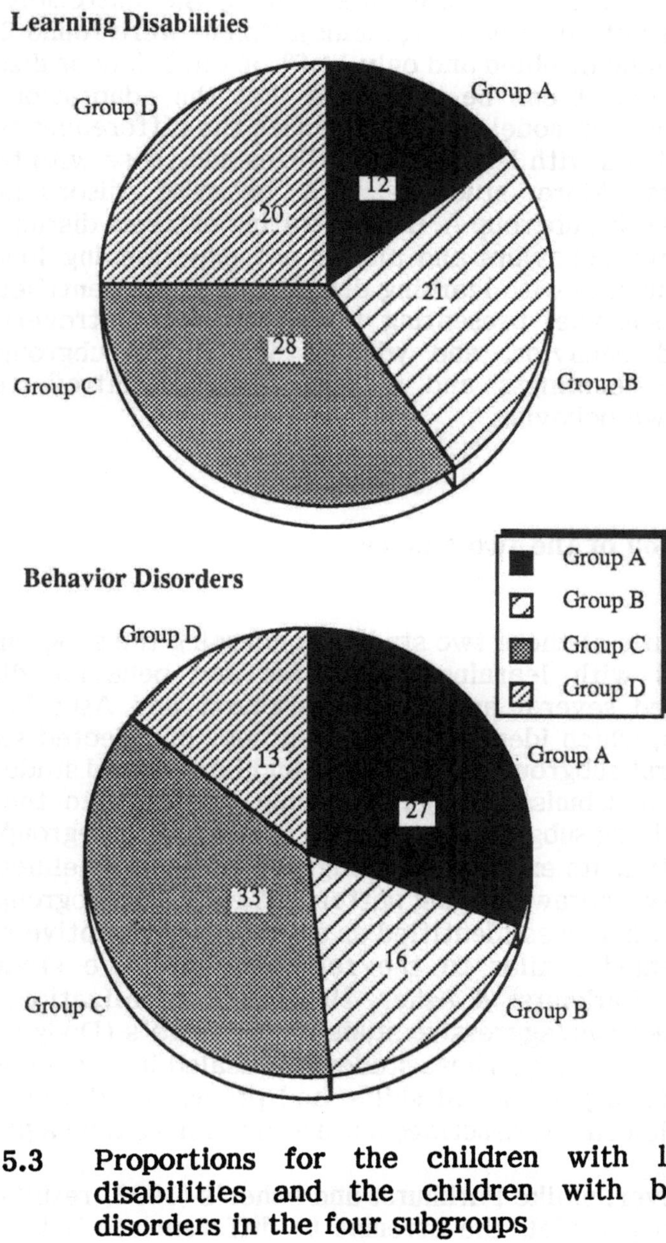

Figure 5.3 Proportions for the children with learning disabilities and the children with behavior disorders in the four subgroups

The largest subgroup was of lonely students with high externalizing maladjustment, in similar proportions for the learning disabled and behavior disordered students. Among the students with behavior disorders, 30% were identified as externalizing non-lonely individuals, compared to only 14.8% of the learning disabled students. Among the extremely lonely students with internalizing maladjustment were found 24.7% of the learning disabled and only 14.6% of the behavior disordered youngsters. It can be concluded that the adaptation of the four-grouping model further clarifies the differences between the students with learning disabilities and those with behavior disorders. More students with behavior disorders were identified in subgroup A, demonstrating extreme disruptive and aggressive behaviors and almost not experiencing loneliness. More students with learning disabilities were identified in the second subtype, presenting relatively more introverted and adjusted behavior, and within the fourth subgroup, with extreme loneliness and a high level of introverted and withdrawn behavior.

Discussion of the two studies

The results of these two studies concerning the subgrouping of students with learning disabilities and behavior disorders resembled several aspects of Parkhurst and Asher's (1992) findings, which identified two subgroups of rejected students. Their first subgroup of withdrawn and introverted students was labeled a submissive-rejected group, similarly to the lonely internalizing subgroup -- subgroup D -- in the four-group model. These students expressed the highest levels of loneliness and a passive-withdrawn coping pattern. The second subgroup in the present study was identified as aggressive, disruptive children and seemed similar to the rejected-aggressive students in Asher's (Parkhurst & Asher, 1992) conceptualization, and to the withdrawn/aggressive students in Dodge's (Dodge & Coie, 1987) terminology. These students revealed impulsive behavior difficulties, poor social skills, and processing deficits. Their aggression can be described more as a reactive than a proactive one.

However, unlike Parkhurst and Asher's (1992) results, in the four-group model, the attempt to differentiate between two subgroups of externalizing students who were high on disruptiveness seems to add an important perspective to understanding the interrelations between disruptive behavior and feelings of loneliness. This differentiation between two subgroups of disruptive students calls for additional research to clarify its interrelations with Landau and Milich's (1985) two-group behavior disorder conceptualization (i.e., solely aggressive and those who have both aggressive and withdrawn tendencies) and with Dodge and Coie's (1987) differentiation between proactive and reactive aggression.

The finding whereby the non-lonely subgroup members with internalizing tendencies were relatively less disruptive in their behavior may account for the inconsistent research results that sometimes failed to identify significant differences between the different clinical categories with mild handicaps. This subgroup should not be ignored, as it further clarifies the complexity of the heterogeneity among groups of children.

The attempt to develop a comprehensive profile of students with learning disabilities and behavior disorders may enhance the understanding of their adjustment difficulties and be valuable in considering multiple processes and behavior within intervention planning. In line with Vaughn and LaGreca's (1992) notion of suiting interventions to students' individual characteristics, and of tailoring interventions to the needs of these students, the proposed model demonstrated the need for comprehensive assessments of behavior profiles in order to apply effective intervention procedures. The efficacy of subtype-to-treatment paradigms requires research and validation, in order to pinpoint the differential effectiveness of various treatment modes for specific subgroups. The subgroups identified in this model may provide a structural prototype for designing intervention planning to meet individual needs and capacities. Future research should evaluate the effectiveness of individually adapted interventions in contrast with more generalized approaches in social skill training.

The process-oriented research for subtype-to-intervention planning may provide additional valuable information, with the goal of emphasizing processes by which individuals with particular subtype profiles learn information and make mistakes, as opposed to research that assesses traits and deficits (McKinney, 1988). The focus of such study lies not on social and academic failure but on learning and processing different types of information -- on the process by which social and academic learning may be successful.

Conclusions

In summary, loneliness appears to be a rather complex phenomenon, with different psychological and behavioral meanings to different individuals within the various subgroups among students with learning disabilities and those with behavior disorders. Whether children respond to loneliness with sadness or aggression, passive withdrawal or active striving for companionship, may depend on personality characteristics, individual histories, and private explanations for loneliness. Environmental conditions and their relations with the subtyping profiles were not examined and still await in-depth study.

To further demonstrate the complex picture, Rothbaum and Weisz (1989) reported that internalizing and externalizing maladjustment behaviors were consistently intermingled, not only in the same child but even in the same episode. Empirical investigations and clinical case studies revealed the strong correlations between internalizing and externalizing scores for most groups of children (Achenbach & Edelbrock, 1983), thus underscoring the need to develop multivariate and dynamic assessments, and to investigate their interrelations with ecological conditions.

Cognitive and emotional realms should both be considered, in order to further our understanding of children's behavior, for example regarding the ability of students with disabilities to read their peers' feelings accurately during social interrelations, to evaluate complex social situations, and to control their behavior. These results may also be studied in relation to the social-information processing of data within the different subgroup members, to understand the social competencies of students with behavior disorders and with learning disabilities, and what contributes to their aggressive retaliation and withdrawal responses. This model suggests that some types of inefficient and inaccurate processing will lead one child to react aggressively in response to conflicts, interpreting peers' intentions as hostile and displaying a greater amount of aggression and retaliation of hostility (Dodge & Coie, 1987). Another child may interpret it differently, behaving in a submissive, withdrawn, and passive pattern. The meaning of aggression for the non-lonely aggressive subgroup is different from that of the lonely aggressive child; it is more instrumental and reinforces itself. The lonely non-aggressive child may feel withdrawn and isolated. This area of research seems promising, yet is in need of extensive research to clarify the theoretical and interventional implications of the developing data base. However, similarly to Landau and Milich's (1985) conclusions, it is clear that valuable information will be lost if, while investigating aggressive and disruptive behaviors, loneliness and withdrawn behavior patterns are not assessed, in order to lead to subtypes and behavior patterns.

Section IV
Coping and Intervention

6 Coping With Loneliness

The unpleasant experience of loneliness for children with and without disabilities can be viewed as a source of stress which individuals try to reduce through different coping activities, according to their unique ways of dealing with difficulties. Virtually every attempt to define social competence has highlighted two main criteria that may also be useful in evaluating the different strategies of coping with loneliness: effectiveness and appropriateness (Guralnick, 1992). Competent behavior implies a high degree of successful outcomes, yet does not exclude a lesser extent of some unsuccessful outcomes. In addition, social competence necessitates acknowledgement and acceptance of the reality that success often includes some forms of compromise or modification of one's original goals.

Effectiveness refers to the availability of a wide repertoire of coping behaviors and the selection of those that will increase the probability of obtaining the desired results. Appropriate social goals and behaviors refer to the age-related norms and standards for interpersonal behavior and friendship networks. Continued use of inappropriate strategies to deal with loneliness and social alienation will have an impact not only on access to groups of peers and individual friends and play partners, but also on the children's own feelings of competency and effective functioning (Guralnick, 1992). Unrealistic expectations for the ultimate social success, such as to be accepted and loved by everybody, without realizing the need for certain compromises, may also affect the child's feelings and behavior.

The study of loneliness and disabilities through children's descriptions of their reactions and behaviors in their attempts to deal effectively and appropriately with their alienation experience may further clarify the construct, and provide valuable information for intervention planning. The coping with stress conceptualization has been used to categorize the behavior descriptions furnished by students with disabilities.

Stress and coping

Loneliness-related stress often leads to ongoing coping responses. Coping can be defined as efforts, both action-oriented (or instrumental) and intrapsychic (or cognitive-emotional), to manage internal and/or external demands which exceed the individual's resources (Folkman, Schaefer, & Lazarus, 1979). Instrumental coping involves direct, problem-oriented actions taken to alter the ongoing person-environment relationship in order to change the stressful situation, whereas cognitive-emotional coping involves a change in the cognitive appraisal of stressors and the emotional reaction to them, with a focus on the regulation of emotion (Antonovsky, 1987; Folkman & Lazarus, 1988). These types of coping responses may be conceptualized as interrelated and as complementing one another within the complex realm of human functioning. Problem-oriented coping refers to efforts to deal with the sources of stress, whether by changing the behavior of the individual or changing the environmental conditions. Emotional regulation refers to coping efforts aimed at reducing emotional distress and maintaining a satisfactory internal state (Coyne & Lazarus, 1981).

Lazarus, one of the leading theoreticians in the conceptualization of coping with stressors, has made major contributions to the conceptual clarification of coping strategies. He viewed coping not as a single, one-dimensional activity or as a structural property of the individual, but rather presented the construct as consisting of a variety of activities aimed toward achieving a change in the environment and/or the individual, within the context of changes across time and in different environments (Folkman & Lazarus, 1988). According to this flexible, ecologically related, and multivariate conceptualization, individuals seem to develop unique patterns of coping strategies that reflect, even within the constant change in behaviors over time and place, a relatively generalized structure that is typical to their unique personality characteristics and cultural and historical environment (Antonovsky, 1979; Holahan & Moos, 1985).

The conceptualization of the interrelations between processes and outcomes of the coping processes (including behavioral and cognitive efforts to deal with the stress) leads to the distinction between more active or approach coping strategies and strategies that rely essentially on avoidance of the problem (Ebata & Moos, 1991; Holahan & Moos, 1985). As discussed in Chapter 3, several studies have pinpointed that active coping was found to be positively related to adjustment, whereas avoidance coping was shown to be related to negative mood and maladjustment (Holahan & Moos, 1985; Margalit & Ankonina, 1991).

Early theory and research undertakings were geared toward identifying independent coping categories that differed in their behavioral reactions. In reality, when faced with stress, most individuals were found to be engaged at the same time in several types of activities: A high level of approach coping may be activated along with different levels of avoidance coping (Holahan & Moos, 1985). Instrumental efforts to change the sources of stress were often accompanied by attempts to modify emotional reactions. Within this multidimensional conceptualization, it is not surprising that adolescents who were identified as having psychological or behavioral problems did not differ from peers on their approach coping, yet were found more likely to respond to stress by using increased amounts of avoidant coping methods, when compared to adolescents without such symptoms (Ebata & Moos, 1991).

Coping efforts which are outer-directed, in order to modify environmental conditions, have often been considered as effectively leading to positive mood (Ebata & Moos, 1991). This concept seems appropriate only when the environment lends itself to change (Margalit, 1990b). In circumstances beyond the individual's control, avoidance coping in terms of efforts to refrain from thinking about the difficulty and to simply accept the negative reality may be considered more adaptive.

Categories for coping with loneliness

In line with the multidimensional and flexible conceptualization of approach and avoidance coping with stress, and based on the response data gathered from different samples of lonely students with and without disabilities who reported how they dealt with their loneliness experience, five categories of activities may be identified (Margalit, 1993a; Parkhurst & Asher, 1992; Rubenstein & Shaver, 1980; Unger, 1992; Woodward & Kalyan-Masih, 1990; Zehavi, 1992). The five types of reactions to the loneliness experience as presented in the different studies were all goal-directed attempts to change the sorrow, pain, and/or anger due to the experience of peer rejection and alienation. The individual's choice of reactions reflects individual differences and a variance in the children's ability to initiate effective and appropriate coping activities. The five coping-with-loneliness responses will be presented with case examples from interviews with children who have mild disabilities (Margalit, 1993a).

A. Sad passivity

Activities characterized as "sad passivity" (Van-Buskirk & Duke, 1991) can be considered to be avoidant coping behaviors. These activities include responses such as crying, oversleeping, sitting, thinking and doing nothing, overeating, and watching television. Interviews with children who have mild disabilities provided examples of sad-passive responses to loneliness:

> *Gil, a 15-year-old male student with learning disabilities, who was fully mainstreamed in a regional junior high school, was described by his teacher as extremely lonely and rated by his peers as rejected. When asked, "What can you do when you feel lonely?" he answered emphatically, "There's nothing you can do, just to be sad."*
>
> *Dana, a 10-year-old female student with reading comprehension difficulties and depressive mood tendencies, was asked to describe what she had done in the past when feeling lonely. She answered, "I went home, went into my room, closed the door after me, and sat in a corner, trying not to cry. After some time I fell asleep."*
>
> *Moshe, a 7-year-old boy with mild mental retardation and attention deficit disorder with hyperactivity who studied in a self-contained special class, described experiencing loneliness: "When it happened I cried and cried, and the time passed so slowly."*
>
> *Ronit, a 16-year-old female student with learning disabilities, reported "I was bored and sad, then I rested in my bed, trying to think how good it could be if I had friends." When the interviewer asked what else she did, she answered "I kept waiting for somebody to come to visit me."*

David, a 9-year-old male student with learning disabilities, was mainstreamed in a regular class during most of the day and received support in a resource classroom for his severe mathematical difficulties. He described a sad-passive response to a loneliness experience: "I was standing near the fence at the corner of the courtyard, looking at the playing children. I thought maybe somebody would notice me and come to talk with me, but nobody came."

Van-Buskirk and Duke (1991), in their study with 33 adolescents, found that the coping style of "sad passivity" was used by lonely and non-lonely adolescents alike, but the non-lonely individuals used this method only temporarily and in preparation of a more active coping style. The potential impact of avoidance and approach strategies depends on their mutual interrelations. According to Roth and Cohen (1986), avoidance and passivity may be regarded as positive coping when they lead to or facilitate and eventually enhance approach coping. The non-lonely youngsters used the coping strategies of a "sad-passive" nature to provide themselves with an opportunity for energizing toward a more active coping. However, lonely individuals appeared to remain in the sad-passive mode for much longer periods (Van-Buskirk & Duke, 1991).

Two considerations may be at work with regard to the relationship between "sad passivity" coping strategies and loneliness. First, the amount of time used for these strategies is important. Second, there may be a hierarchy of strategies in which individuals engage when responding to loneliness, that may be tied to situational factors yet also may be in line with Rook and Peplau's (1982) suggestion regarding the need for some quiet time prior to active coping. Van-Buskirk and Duke (1991) suggested that there may even be times when sad-passive strategies are temporarily adaptive, such as when the youngster needs time to get over strong feelings of anger and frustration before being able to actively socialize with peers.

B. Active search for social contacts and friends

In this category, efforts are focused at creating and extending social contacts through the use of approach or active coping behaviors. Children's activities are directed at changing their actual social relations by forming new relationships or by using the existing network more fully. This type of coping involves the initiation of activities through behaviors such as calling a peer on the telephone, visiting someone, or trying to meet new children at the local community center. Similarly to Carver, Scheier, and Weintraub's (1989) conceptualization of active coping, in this category the individual is taking active steps in an attempt to remove the stressor or ameliorate its effects. Active coping includes increasing one's efforts and initiating direct actions to change the social situation. To facilitate goals such as raising one's self-esteem and reputation within the children's group, children reported activities such as:

> *"doing something that you're good at, like bringing a skateboard or a ball, riding on a bike"*
> or
> *"inviting children to play with your computer games."*

Interview material from children with mild disabilities (Margalit, 1993a) exemplifies this category of active coping responses to experiences of loneliness and social isolation:

> *Shari, a 13-year-old female student with behavior disorders, aggressive behavior, and a low tolerance for frustration, reported: "When I moved into a new school, I went over to a group of children - boys and girls - and began talking with them, telling them my name. Saying - I am new here."*

> *Avi, a 7-year-old boy with learning disabilities and behavior difficulties, described, "I felt lonely and bored in the afternoons. I knew that all my classmates were playing and having fun, but I am alone a lot in school. One afternoon, nobody came to see me, and I didn't have anything to do. So, I took my new ball, went downstairs, and started playing by myself. Sure enough, some kids gathered around, looking at me. I invited them to play with me, saying that even though my ball was new and pretty expensive, we could still play together with it. They liked my offer. I could see that some of them were younger than my classmates, in the first grade, but I didn't care."*

> *Baruch, an 11-year-old boy with reading and spelling difficulties, reported, "I asked my brother to take me with*

him when he went to play with friends, even though they were two years younger - and he was not very happy to do it."

Mira, a 10-year-old female student with learning disabilities and language difficulties, said, "I went to friends, to their homes. I didn't call them on the telephone, but went to visit them. I hoped that they also had nothing better to do, and would be happy to play with me."

Avraham, a 13-year-old boy with mild mental retardation, described: "I saw some boys that I hadn't met before, who were playing in the yard near my house, and I talked with them. I asked them if I could join their game."

These descriptions represent the children's active attempts to find friends, to extend their companionship networks, and to avoid periods at school or in the afternoons when the children found themselves alone. The coping methods focused on the initiation of activities and on the use of games and ideas to persuade children to develop relationships and join in play activities. These efforts revealed the children's willingness to compromise by seeking less desirable companionship (especially younger children), in order to play with somebody. Some of these efforts were successful, fostering the attainment of the desired goals. Yet others ended in disappointments, rejection, and feeling used. Several children reported incidents such as:

"They agreed to play with my ball [or with my new computer games], but after an hour they left me. I could see them playing outside without inviting me to go on playing with them."

C. Active solitary activities

Children develop alternative solitary activities in order to stay busy and avoid the loneliness experience (Rubenstein & Shaver, 1980). This category includes such responses as exercising, studying, and working; reading and writing; listening to music, watching television programs, walking, running, swimming; working on a hobby; and going to a movie. These activities represent active efforts to change the individual's social needs or desires, through a widening of the repertoire of tasks and activities that are undertaken and that are viewed as enjoyable and satisfying yet can be performed alone. This approach type of coping does not strive to change the children's actual social relations. It concentrates on the children's internal processing, aiming to cognitively redefine their problem by differentiating between the experience of staying alone and feelings of loneliness. Many children with disabilities (Margalit, 1993a) reported that they spend much time in activities such as playing different games alone (e.g., computer games); doing arts and crafts such as painting; putting music on very loudly; and helping with the household chores. They were even able to conclude that *"thinking about other things"* and *"keeping busy at home"* may help when feeling lonely.

Computer games and activities may be seen as a solitary activity that can play an important role for children with disabilities. The entrance of home-computing (Margalit, 1990a) into the repertoire of activities of children with and without disabilities has the potential of initiating change in their family climate, or of supporting the existing dynamic among the family members. Margalit (1991c) found that within a group of students with learning disabilities, loneliness experience was predicted not only by peer acceptance levels and social skills, but also by their attitudes toward using computers within their repertoire of free-time activities at home. The more these students were accepted by peers, viewed themselves as socially competent, and also found computer activities to be enjoyable, the lower their loneliness feelings.

D. Asking for help

In order to avoid the loneliness experience, the help of peers or adults may be requested. Acknowledging the reality that they have not been successful at changing their social situation by themselves, children may approach peers or adults for assistance. Several children who used this coping method asked classmates to call them when they go to the local youth club. Others approached adults such as teachers, counselors, and parents, sharing with them how lonely they felt and expecting them to help or support their efforts to find playmates (Margalit, 1993a).

The request for help may be manifested either as a direct approach activity, where the child expresses an expectation that the help-provider will give assistance in finding a friend, or as a less direct approach activity, where consultation or advice is sought in terms of "How can I...?" Sometimes the lonely child may feel secure enough to disclose that he or she is lonely, and at other times, the major focus of complaint may be boredom, described as: *"I have nothing to do and no friends to play with."*

E. Aggressive, disruptive behaviors

Several children described how they acted out their anger, annoyance, and frustration through aggressiveness and disruptiveness, when experiencing loneliness and rejection by peers (Margalit, 1993a):

> *Roni, a 6-year-old developmental delayed boy with speech difficulties, said "I hit and cursed the boys when they didn't want me to play with them and told me to go away and leave them alone."*

> *Avner, a 16-year-old male student with behavior difficulties, told of one incident where he used aggressive coping mechanisms: "He didn't want me to play with him or his friends. I was so lonely, angry and hurt. I had nothing to do, nothing to lose. So I went over and let the air out of the tire of his bicycle, yelled at him, and then I ran away."*

> *Gila, a 10-year-old learning disabled female student with attention deficient disorder, told the school counselor: "It makes you crazy to see everybody having fun, and not wanting me in the group. I feel alone and angry, so I throw their books to the floor, and the teacher gets angry at me. Nobody understands me."*

These children and adolescents reported on their extremely angry and painful feelings that lead to disruptive and uncontrolled aggression. At times, their aggressiveness seemed connected to a sense of hopelessness, and their lack of attempts to concentrate efforts on controlling their anger was justified by their hopeless feeling of having nothing to lose.

Surveys on the usage of coping-with-loneliness strategies

Categories based on interview data among 80 male students with learning disabilities from grades 2 to 8 in three cities in Israel (Unger, 1992; Zehavi, 1992) illustrated their coping activities. Figure 6.1 demonstrates the proportions of the five different types of coping activities in an attempt to end their experience of loneliness, as reported by the children themselves. As presented in the figure, students with learning disabilities were engaged in two major coping activities that both seemed to express acceptance of their social isolation: sad-passive activities (avoidance coping) and alternative-solitary activities (approach coping with a focus on activities that can be performed alone, and activation of internal processing). Most of these students felt that they could not develop satisfying social interrelations, and either accepted this fact and tried to develop satisfying activities to fill their free time and replace their social needs, or else stayed alone and felt sorry for themselves.

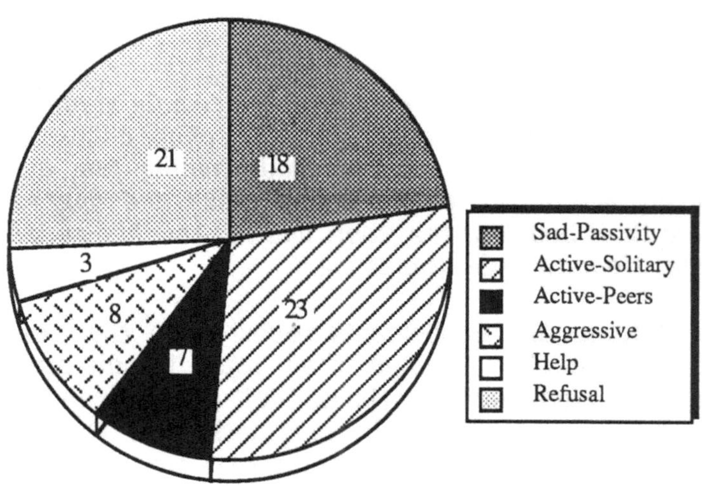

Figure 6.1 Proportions of students with learning disabilities in the categories for coping with loneliness

Only a few students attempted to directly change their social situation, either through active performance (searching for a friend and even being ready to compromise by playing with younger students) or asking for the help of a peer or adult. According to students' self-reports, only 10% were engaged in aggressive or disruptive activities following their loneliness experience. It is not clear if teachers' and parents' perceptions will support this report by children as to their coping responses to the experience of loneliness, or to what extent the interview findings may represent the children's individual perceptions or even their defensive trends. It should be emphasized that a relatively high proportion of the lonely students (1/5 of the samples) refused to answer the question about what they did when felt lonely. About half of them declared in a most defensive manner that they do not remember even once feeling lonely. Although the use of avoidance strategies may be adaptive in certain situations and at certain stages of the coping process, persistent reliance on these types of responses, particularly with chronic social difficulties with peers, may prove costly for long-term adjustment (Ebata & Moos, 1991).

Individualized coping style

The categorization of activities that children performed to deal with their experience of loneliness seemed closely related to individual differences, in both the range of the preferred activities and the personal meaning that the child attributed to them. Research demonstrated that relatively stable individual differences were found in the amount of time that individuals spent alone (Csikszentmihalyi & Larson, 1984). Furthermore, decreased social activity and increased active engagement in solitary activities were found to be two independent dimensions and not to be on a continuum (Csikszentmihalyi & Larson, 1984). Some children can be very active in both social-interpersonal and solitary activities, whereas others may remain inactive in both and complain of boredom.

Television watching was reported as one of the most popular activities for lonely students, yet its meaning seemed to vary among the children. Moore and Schultz (1983) found a significant correlation between levels of loneliness among adolescents and watching television. Students who reported feeling more lonely watched television for longer periods of time. Luftig (1987) also found that television watching was related in children's reports to feelings of social incompetence. However, several children with disabilities when interviewed reported not only that they spent much time watching television, but that they found this time to be very enjoyable. They suggested that when they had nothing else to do, this was a preferred activity. Thus, watching television for children with disabilities may be considered as a solitary alternative activity, although it may also be regarded as a passive activity, requiring careful investigation of the child's interpretations and attributions.

Computer activities may be regarded both as an age-appropriate solitary alternative activity and as a manifestation of active efforts to expand one's group activities. Playing computer games has been widely depicted as one of the most preferred activities of disabled and nondisabled children alike, both in the home and at school (Margalit, 1990a). Computer games and simulations are attractive and challenging, and they stimulate curiosity and fantasy. Solitary computer activities, especially computer games, may be considered extremely valuable for lonely children as an independent yet pleasurable means for filling unstructured leisure time. Solitary computer play may assist these youngsters in distracting themselves from self-pity and angry thoughts and at the same time also in developing an area of competence that may foster self-esteem and be used at a later stage as a basis for expanding companionship relations. However, individual differences were noticed between youngsters who developed an "addiction" to solitary computer games and continued to play alone, and those youngsters who, with renewed motivation after periods of solitary activity, actively utilized their new competency as a basis for new social relations.

Both computer games and television watching can be used by lonely children as solitary activities to fill their leisure time. The children's ability to exploit these activities for enhancing peer relations depends on their level of motivation to pursue social interactions. An examination of the motivation of lonely students highlights contradictory trends reflecting individual differences. On the one hand, among some lonely children, their strong wish to have friends leads them toward initiating social interactions and avoiding situations where there is a great probability of remaining alone. For example:

Gur, a 10-year-old boy with learning disabilities, said convincingly "You should do everything, give them your ball, let them win, tell them your secrets, and even be ready to play with younger children -- but don't stay alone."

On the other hand, loneliness among other children was described as related to a decrease in motivation necessary to focus efforts on creating a change in social relations. Sometimes children described their experience as one of paralyzing hopelessness, fatigue, and lack of strength. In our interviews, several children gave responses such as:

"When you're lonely you can't do anything. You're better off just going home and closing the door of your room behind you."

These contradictory motivational trends may reflect either different types of loneliness (social and emotional loneliness, with emotional loneliness more related to reduced motivation), different personality subtyping (externalizing versus internalizing loneliness), different coping strategies, and/or different stages in the experience of loneliness. The longer an individual experiences loneliness, the less his or her efforts will be channeled into changing this reality.

Attempts to categorize coping-with-loneliness strategies through research have indicated that the full meaning attributed by the children to their loneliness and coping activities can only be understood by evaluating the children's disabling conditions, their subjective levels of distress, well-being, and resilience, and the contextual conditions in which the behavior was performed. Single activities cannot be assumed to reflect the child's response pattern to loneliness experiences. Only the simultaneous consideration of all of an individual student's emotional reactions and coping behaviors can clarify their interdependence and relative meaning for that student (Ebata & Moos, 1991).

Context-related coping behaviors: Two examples

Two types of behavior will be used to exemplify the complexity and interdependence of the strategies' meaning within the context of the social environment:

1 Entry behavior among preschool children
2 Self-disclosure behavior among school-age children

Entry strategies in a preschool environment

The following are two examples of preschool children's behavior when seeking to enter a social group.

> *Gidon, a 4-year-old boy, arrived late to his class. He could see some of the boys he liked engaged in play with blocks and cars in the activity corner of the nursery school. He quickly went over to them, but they continued to play and plan their game aloud, ignoring him. He stood quietly next to them, listened carefully for a few minutes, and then brought over a bigger block from the corner. He held it in his hands and suggested, "You need a bridge for your cars to get home." One of the children answered rejectingly, "We don't want your bridge." Yet a second child said, "Put the bridge next to the tall building, not where you are standing." Gidon did not argue, although initially he had wanted to put the block in another location. Soon he became a partner in the game, suggesting new ideas, arguing about car locations, and interacting as if he had been a member of the group from the beginning.*

> *Rami, a 5-year-old developmental delayed boy, whose sensori-motor coordination difficulties resulted in clumsiness, observed some of the popular boys playing with blocks and cars. He ran happily towards them, shouting "me too." They then defensively said "don't touch." They called the teacher for help, saying, "Take him away - he'll destroy everything." Rami began crying and promised to stand by quietly and watch. The teacher let him stay, but did not ask the group to let him participate in the game. After a few quiet minutes, he took a block and said "Look at me - I can do it," trying to add his block to the top of one of the block-buildings. All of the children in the group began shouting together, telling him to go somewhere else and calling the teacher to have her remove him from the area.*

These two descriptions focus attention on one of the most critical, difficult, and complex tasks that children face from the early stages of socialization: to discover how to join and become involved in peer activities such as play that are already ongoing, while aiming to avoid feelings of loneliness. Researchers were interested in how young children approach and strive to enter into the ongoing activities of groups of their peers (Putallaz & Wasserman, 1990). Because successful initiation of entry into the peer play group is a prerequisite for further social interactions, whereas unsuccessful entry performance may lead to feelings of rejection and loneliness, this behavior can be considered as a major, complicated task that children face at the preschool stage.

It is tempting to assume that one of the typical characteristics of socially rejected and lonely children is their failure in entry behavior. However, it appears that about 50% of all initial attempts to enter a group by children of different levels of social status are rejected or ignored by peers (Guralnick, 1992). Those children who succeed in joining a group must develop a series of strategies and skills and learn to select the ones that will help persuade their companions to allow them to participate in the group's activities. Several basic skills are needed to enable the successful entry into an ongoing group activity:

1. *Persistence*. To overcome rejection, children must learn to persist in their attempts to enter the group.

2. *Understanding the group activity*. Cognitive difficulties may cause children to misjudge the group behavior and to use mistaken behaviors as a key to seeking entry.

3. *Controlling impulsive behavior*. Self-control is essential to enable the child to observe and listen before attempting to enter the group, in order to suggest relevant activities and contents and to prevent disruptive behavior that may incite rejection.

4. *Alternative activities*. Children must exhibit a willingness and the ability to propose alternative activities in the face of initial failure.

The child's capacity to accurately perceive the ongoing group activity constitutes a central strategy for group entry. Appropriate understanding and judgment of what is happening in the group enables the child to select relevant remarks and to behave adaptively, thus promoting his/her acceptance into the group by developing harmony with the group's activity rather than being intrusive. Gidon, for instance, first attended to the group quietly, attempting to understand what the children were undertaking. His suggestion to introduce a bridge was well integrated into the group's activity.

On the other hand, self-statements or comments that tend to redirect the children's ongoing activities may lead to peer rejection (Guralnick, 1992). Children with disabilities were found to employ more entry strategies that brought the attention of the group to themselves, such as self-focused statements or disruptions of the group activity (Putallaz & Wasserman, 1990). The degree of intrusiveness also appears to have a clear impact on the success of entry trials, where less intrusive and less direct strategies (e.g., producing a variant of ongoing behavior) facilitate entrance into the group. The impulsiveness of many disabled children may be perceived by the group as intrusiveness, thus leading to rejection and denial of entrance into the group's activity.

Children with disabilities may encounter specific difficulties in controlling their impulsive temperament in order to analyze social information from the group and to attend patiently to peers' communications. Their cognitive and perceptual difficulties may impede the ability to obtain sufficient and accurate information that will enable an understanding of the interactions between the children, in order to select an appropriate entry behavior. Processing the information available from the play context is critical in order to select the appropriate entry strategy.

Dodge (1986) has developed a model of social-cognitive processing as related to social tasks. The model may elucidate the required competencies that may be deficient among children with disabilities. Within this model, it is hypothesized that children process social information in five sequential steps:

1. Encoding social cues in the present situation
2. Mentally representing and interpreting those cues
3. Generating possible behavioral responses (strategies)
4. Evaluating the consequences of possible responses and selecting a specific strategy
5. Enacting a behavioral response

All of these steps are important to ensure effective entry behavior, and cognitive and non-cognitive difficulties may occur at one or more of the steps in this sequential process. Children with disabilities can be expected to exhibit deficits in several of these steps, thus failing to adequately process social information.

Conflict resolution strategies

Another critical aspect of the peer entry situation relates to the strategies that children employ to resolve conflicts. Although persistence is a necessary condition for group entrance, considering the high rate of expected rebuffs, persistent attempts to enter into group activities may lead to conflicts. Thus, the means used by children to select and organize strategies in order settle conflicts constitute important skills for promoting acceptance by the group. Strategies for conflict resolution include negotiation, compromise, and making alternative suggestions (Hazen & Black, 1989). Gidon, for example, did not try to rigidly force his concept on the group (i.e., he agreed to change the place of the bridge according to one peer's suggestion), and he showed persistence but did not enter into a quarrel with the one child who actively tried to reject him.

Children in conflictual situations may insist or even threaten other children. They may offer counter proposals or express a readiness for reaching compromises. When arguing, they may or may not provide reasons for their actions. Insight into the ways in which conflicts are managed effectively among peers may illuminate the paths to success or failure of the bid for entry, underscoring the variation in strategies among individual children and along different situations and times.

In addition, the child's social status and "reputation" within the group will also affect peers' processing of his/her entry behavior. Behaviors, even mistakes, of popular and accepted children will be judged differently from those of socially rejected peers. Putallaz and Wasserman (1990) concluded in their research survey that the ineffective entry behavior exhibited by low-status or rejected children may be related to their greater concern for "saving face" when confronted with peers' negative responses, but also leads at the same time to further rejection and isolation. Peers will evaluate these children's behavior using less accepting and understanding attitudes and will view their mistakes as providing justification for their initial rejection. Thus the complexity of the use of entry coping strategies may be understood only within the complex social situation, even at early stages of socialization.

Self-disclosure in the school environment

Another area of research -- in self-disclosure -- may exemplify the complexity of behavior among lonely individuals in their efforts to cope with their loneliness. Self-disclosure strategies demonstrate the varying degrees of control that individuals maintain over their own personal and private information (Derlega & Margulis, 1982), as related to the goals they want to achieve through its regulation. Self-disclosure to peers (and not to parents) was considered to be associated with less loneliness and more intimate social interrelations (Solano, Batten, & Parish, 1982). Several lonely students with disabilities suggested that an effective way to develop close companionship is through sharing secrets (Margalit, 1993a). Derlega and Margulis (1982) identified four major goals for self-disclosure behavior:

1 *Expressive functions.* Instead of bottling up distressed feelings, the child is able to speak about his/her difficulties, and the activity is used for emotional ventilation.

2 *Relationship development.* The sharing of personal secrets and the communication of private issues are used to express special trust, intimacy, and closeness in order to enhance friendships.

3 *Self-clarification.* Children reveal their private affairs to ensure that their behavior is correctly understood by peers. When their communications have enabled the identification of a misunderstanding, children may further disclose their intentions and activities.

4 *Social validation.* Children share personal information in order to obtain the feedback and reactions that comprise social norms and clarify social attitudes.

Self-disclosure behavior and loneliness were found to be linked among high school students (Davis & Franzoi, 1986). An increase in self-disclosure behavior with peers was negatively related to feelings of loneliness. It may be understood that the more an individual shares private matters and uses self-disclosure as a coping strategy, the less he or she feels lonely. However, an alternative perspective cannot be ignored, which views loneliness tendencies as a personality disposition that is also responsible for a tendency toward withdrawal, retaining distance, and reduced levels of self-disclosure, as discussed in Chapter 2.

Self-consciousness produces disclosure, which in turn reduces loneliness. The tendency to share private information with one's peers is associated with one's own tendency to be engaged in a state of self-awareness and with one's motivation for intimate relations (Franzoi & Davis, 1985). The possibility should also be considered that individuals who are low in self-consciousness feel reluctant to engage in activities in which personal, possibly intense and sometimes even negative feelings may be felt and expressed. Awareness of the relations between mood and personal concerns introduces an additional dimension to the complexity of the phenomena, highlighting the fact that increased attention to private self-aspects appears to intensify the affective charge of moods (Greenberg & Musham, 1981). It is possible that individuals who are low in private self-consciousness may attempt to avoid engaging in private self-awareness and self-disclosure partly in order to avoid this intensification of affect that frightens them.

Self-disclosure and disabilities

The study of friendship relations among individuals with developmental disabilities (Clegg & Standen, 1991) revealed that most of these individuals had relatively superficial interrelations with friends that were not characterized by sharing of more personal concerns. The descriptive construct of these friendships was similar to a description of relations with strangers in nondisabled individuals. The low self-disclosure among disabled students may be related to their low self-esteem, defensive attitudes, and reluctance to expose private matters (Bolea, 1986). However, it is unclear whether this tendency revealed their inner insecurity, distrust, and fear of revealing difficulties, or whether the self-disclosure may be related to limited communicative abilities or a deficit or delay in the ability for self-observation. Clinical observations have indicated that these individuals often communicate loneliness experiences and desires for friendships in an immature style.

More research is needed to explore the sources of the limited age-appropriate self-disclosure behavior and to analyze in detail what types of self-disclosure may be considered to be effective strategies for dealing with loneliness and what types may represent maladaptive or immature coping strategies that lead to further peer rejection, loneliness, and alienation.

A focus on the lower self-disclosure behavior evidenced by aggressive children may enhance the full understanding of this phenomenon. Many aggressive children were found to report a strong need to present themselves positively to others, creating a tendency to establish more superficial interpersonal relations (Epanchin & Rennells, 1989). These findings may be understood as related to difficulties in cognitive and emotional regulation of strong feelings, resulting in powerful defensive tendencies. The restricted self-disclosure behavior may thereby express an attempt to deny feelings that the child may fear will be considered by peers as negative, undesirable, and inappropriate.

Conclusions

In conclusion, the study of children's strategies to cope with loneliness experiences underscored that these activities can be identified in isolation only for methodological purposes. In reality they represent complex behaviors whose effectiveness and appropriateness can be evaluated only within their specific contexts of time and place. The same behaviors can be used by the lonely and the non-lonely child to achieve different goals. The adaptive orientation in stress research has fostered a growing interest in stress resistance, with an emphasis on the value of effective coping strategies (Holahan & Moos, 1990). Individual differences, personal vulnerability, and resilience have been conceptualized as developing from the effective and noneffective confrontation with stressful experiences through adaptive emotional and behavioral coping, leading to positive psychosocial growth (Holahan & Moos, 1990). Children react to the stress of their loneliness using various types of active and avoidance coping strategies, and their adaptive or maladaptive value may be judged only with reference to the child's individual differences and the environmental expectations and standards. Two behaviors -- entrance into groups and self-disclosure -- were used to exemplify the complexity of the construct. Appropriateness and effectiveness, as two criteria used to judge coping strategies, can serve as a guide to intervention planning.

7 Approaches in Intervention Research

In this chapter, the results of the intervention research and major conclusion issues that were found significant in the intervention and training of social competence will be presented, with the objective of clarifying their implications for planning effective intervention programs to promote effective coping with the loneliness experience. In the first part of this chapter, a brief overview of research surveys on social skills training will be presented as related to models and their specific contents and procedures, in order to highlight their principal conclusions having strong relevance for planning loneliness interventions. In the second part, the implications of these programs for loneliness intervention research will be specified.

Conclusions from prior interventions

The study of loneliness in children with disabilities is new, and intervention research with a focus on this subject is at its initial stages. However, an extensive body of intervention research has already explored the social competence and adaptive behavior of children with mild disabilities. Comprehensive surveys (Andrasik & Matson, 1985; Bryan & Lee, 1990; Coie, 1985; Coie & Koeppl, 1990; Hansen, Watson-Perczel, & Christopher, 1989; Jupp & Griffiths, 1990; Ladd & Asher, 1985; LaGreca & Santogrossi, 1980; Mize & Ladd, 1990; Oden & Asher, 1977; Pellegrini & Urbain, 1985; Vaughn & LaGreca, 1992) have revealed the different levels of positive impact demonstrated by various studies, thus alerting intervention planners to the limited value of simplistic models and emphasizing several crucial issues necessary to promote intervention programs' success.

Hansen, Watson-Perczel, and Christopher (1989) surveyed research on social skills training of adolescents with a variety of difficulties of an externalizing nature (e.g., aggressiveness, delinquency, behavior disorders) and of an internalizing nature (e.g., withdrawal, shyness). Clinical groups such as adolescents with emotional difficulties or with mental retardation were also included. They reported that these research investigations in general have provided support for the effectiveness of social-interaction interventions with adolescents. Studies in Coie and Koeppl's (1990) survey revealed that social skills training has had a positive effect on social behavior, as translated into actual improvement in social acceptance by peers, linking skills improvement to gains in sociometric data.

Other research surveys revealed less consistent findings. In a number of studies (LaGreca & Santogrossi, 1980) using different measures for assessment, inconsistent findings were demonstrated. An increase in knowledge regarding adaptive behavior was evident in some of these studies, yet no change was found for the children's acceptance measure. Other studies (Oden & Asher, 1977) reported increased peer acceptance, although post-test observations did not reveal significant behavior differences in social interactions. Interventions for preschool children (Mize & Ladd, 1990) revealed an increase in acceptance scores measured after a one-month follow-up interval, but aggressive behavior did not decrease. Oden and Asher (1977) found that children who received social skill training (in cooperation, communication, etc.) displayed long-term improvement in peer status but not in friendship networking. In can be concluded that the results of intervention research pinpointed the importance of the different models, samples, and contextual conditions in predicting the effectiveness of interventions.

Social intervention models: Deficit and systemic approaches

Two major approaches were developed in order to promote the social competence of children with disabilities:

1 The deficit model, with a focus on the target child with disabilities and social difficulties, in order to directly change his/her skills.
2 The systemic model, with a global focus on the system and its parts, in order to change the environmental climate.

Deficit models

The first approach underlying social skills interventions views the disabling condition itself -- the lack or delay in critical skills for positive social interactions -- as the root of these children's difficulties. Poorer social interactions are seen according to this approach as a consequence and not as the basic problem. Within the deficit model (Asher & Renshaw, 1981), children who lack age-appropriate social skills will experience social difficulties and will acquire a poorer social status among their peers. Most social skill training programs with an underlying deficit model have attempted to identify skills that are considered critical for the growth of competent social functioning and use instruction strategies for low-status children.

Mize and Ladd (1990) proposed a social skill model that can be adapted to different age groups of children. This model suggested that in order for children to act in a socially skilled manner, they must (a) possess social knowledge of goals and contexts; (b) be able to translate knowledge into skilled performance; and (c) continuously monitor and evaluate their environment and their impact on contextual conditions. Within this conceptualization, children's difficulties may stem from deficient processing of environmental interactions, from performance difficulties, and/or from faulty monitoring due to a failure in evaluating the processing of social interactions.

Every social skills training program based on the deficit model must define the two major issues of contents (i.e., defining the crucial social skills) and procedures (i.e., defining the preferred strategies to acquire these skills).

Content selection: Critical skills

Any working model for intervention planning requires the selection of those skills critical for ensuring age-related social competence and effective coping with loneliness. Two approaches to skill selection have been used: one generalized and the other specialized (Ladd, 1981). The generalized approach aims to increase the proportion of age-related adaptive behaviors for the children with deficient social processing, through the training and enhancing of many prosocial skills, without explicitly aspiring to focus training on specific social skills or to directly link the identified difficulties or specific training contents. The more specialized approach seeks to identify specific areas of need and difficulty and to train the child in these deficient areas. Within the second approach, the social validation of the trained skills should be carefully examined (Hansen, Watson-Perczel, & Christopher, 1989) and assessed individually as related to context. It should be emphasized that even with regard to theoretically valid skills for competent social behavior, moderate to high amounts of variance have been demonstrated within the range of competent functioning, reflecting personal style.

Children's social style may differ in several important aspects, such as the size of their social network, levels of self-disclosure, extent of involvement in social activities, and stylistic behavioral components (e.g., eye contact, response relevance, response timing). Groups of children also have different styles and norms that define their peers' social competence, such as appearance (the way they dress and talk), communication style (the way they ask questions or ask for help), and their conflict resolution patterns. Context-related specific social validation may be established through a survey of peer ratings within the specific group to which the target children belong. In one study (Hansen, Watson-Perczel, & Christopher, 1989), children were asked with whom they would like to play within their peer group. Then these children were asked to provide descriptions of the behaviors of those peers with whom they prefer to play. The discrepancies between the descriptions of ideal playmates and of the target children were used to select the skills to be developed through intervention.

Different specific skills have been identified in various programs and reports as the goals for specialized intervention approaches. Plienis, Hansen, Ford, and Smith (1987) reported on an intervention with a group of emotionally handicapped teenagers who were considered deficient in their communication efficiency and problem solving abilities. This program, focusing on training in conversation skills and social problem solving, resulted in improved self-esteem, higher teacher ratings of adjustment, and decreased loneliness.

Oden and Asher (1977) viewed four skills as the most important for promoting the social competence of third and fourth graders: cooperation with peers and adults, participation in group activities, communication using clear messages, and supportiveness of one another. In another study, the goals of intervention were to foster children's participation and group involvement through advancing these deficient four skills (Coie & Koeppl, 1990).

The core of Ladd's (1981) intervention comprised three verbal social skills that demonstrated the children's difficulties and were considered critical for competent social behavior. The first skill was asking questions in a friendly manner as a means for initiating and maintaining social interaction. The second skill was making positive suggestions to peers in terms of initiating, elaborating, maintaining, and offering support for joint play and activities. The third social skill, commenting (e.g., saying frequently what they are doing), was expected to help peers define common goals by adding suggestions and comments.

It can be concluded that, in various programs, the general and the specific skills both dealt with similar areas of social functioning yet emphasized some of them differently. Most of the programs concerned the promotion of cooperation, group involvement, and communication -- with a differential focus on asking questions, making suggestions, commenting, verbal reinforcements, and peer supportiveness. The programs differed not only in the specific target skills within the different categories, but also in their procedure of instruction and training.

Procedure selection: Preferred strategies

A three-stage sequence was suggested by many social skill training programs.

Stage I. The first stage gears efforts toward the effective instruction of the new skill. The modeling and coaching approaches often used in the instruction of skills seem promising for teaching complex social behaviors. Modeling strategies teach skills by demonstrating competent performance in specific social behaviors. Coaching strategies explicitly provide the principles of competent social behavior, usually with behavioral examples. The learner is expected to use the general principle to generate appropriate social behaviors in different contexts and situations (Pellegrini & Urbain, 1985). Gresham and Nagle (1980) compared coaching, modeling, and a combined coaching-modeling procedure and compared them to a "no treatment" group. In the modeling procedure, a group of children viewed videotapes of interactions between youngsters and, with adult guidance, discussed the behaviors and skills presented. In the coaching procedure, a group received adult instruction and an opportunity for active performance, rehearsal, and experimentation of the learned skills and behaviors instead of passive attendance to the films. Both conditions included active adult instruction and were found effective, with the combined coaching-modeling procedure as most effective.

The problem solving approach has served as a prototype for a variety of intervention programs. These interventions used procedures for instructing methods such as alternative thinking -- generating multiple solutions to a problem situation; consequential thinking -- the ability to consider the short- and long-term consequences of activities; and means-end thinking -- the ability to plan a series of actions to reach a specific goal (Shure & Spivack, 1978, 1979). Attention is directed toward enhancing self-regulating skills such as checking, planning, monitoring, testing, and evaluating solutions to difficulties (e.g., to "plan" how to initiate communication; to "monitor" their support of peers) (Borkowski, Day, Saenz, Dietmeyer, Estrada, & Groteluschen, 1992; Swanson, 1990).

Stage II. The goal of the second stage is to promote skilled performance. The procedures in this stage include rehearsing and exercising, to increase the students' access to the solutions and behaviors already acquired. This stage of training involves: (a) providing the learner with opportunities for guided rehearsal, and rehearsing in a sheltered context; (b) evaluating the performance of the learner by providing feedback comparing standards and performance, to enhance feelings of self-efficacy in the learner; and (c) fostering skill elaboration through skill reformulation and elaboration.

Stage III. The third stage endeavors to foster maintenance and generalization by assisting the learner to become independent in the performance of the new skill, so as to continue performing it in varied settings and for a long period after the training is concluded. This goal may be accomplished by (a) providing opportunities for self-directed rehearsal, (b) encouraging self-initiation of performance while withdrawing performance cues or aids, and (c) fostering self-evaluation by promoting self-monitoring.

Maintenance has been targeted in several programs through the continuation of intervention until mastery of the skill has been attained. The construction of a system of booster sessions, consisting of short training periods following a specified period without training, will facilitate skill maintenance (Lochman, 1985, 1988). Generalization to other settings, other individuals, and over time should be targeted and planned. The generalization of treatment effects can be assessed for the use of social skills with novel persons, novel situations or problems, and different settings than the trained one (Haring & Liberty, 1990). Special value should be attributed to the assessment of relationships with peers within natural environments (Hansen, Watson-Perczel, & Christopher, 1989). Generalization can occur spontaneously after skill acquisition, but most often it does not, requiring careful and detailed programming to promote performance (Haring & Liberty, 1990).

Systemic models

A second group of studies has proposed a systemic approach to social intervention, highlighting the children's environmental conditions at home or school and focusing on the interrelations between the child's functioning and these conditions. From the systemic perspective, Vaughn, McIntosh, and Hogan (1990) viewed the deficit model of social relations as inadequate because it fails to address important components of social relationships, environmental influences, and their ongoing interactions. A deficit model assumes that the problem is within the child and that the target for change is the child himself or herself.

The systemic model assumes that individual relationships can be understood only within the social-structural context. Social skills training programs are considered a potential part of the systemic model, but not as sufficient to alter social status independently. This approach is based on the assumption that a high probability exists that children whose development was delayed and who experienced repeated failures in several areas of functioning will be more rejected by peers and will interact differently and infrequently with them. Thus, children with disabilities may be deprived of age-appropriate opportunities to learn new skills and to exercise them until the point of mastery (Coie & Koeppl, 1990), and individuals in these systems (peers, teachers, parents, and/or siblings) will develop unique interactional patterns with the children that may further enhance their difficulties.

The goals of systemic interventions are to increase and reinforce the children's frequency of successful interactions with peers and adults. Systemic changes are expected to develop conditions in the environment that will promote positive social interactions and group involvement, enhancing friendship networks, social identity, and support, and decreasing aggressive and disruptive behavior.

Accepting the assumption that the lack of age-appropriate social experiences is the root of the difficulties among children with disabilities, systemic interventions are directed at behaviors and attitudes leading toward companionship and avoiding loneliness. Intervention planning according to this approach targets those contents and procedures that will be directed not toward the individuals with deficiencies and difficulties, but rather toward the development of an environment that enables, enhances, and reinforces social interactions. This environment promotes social interactions in terms of:

1 Positive yet realistic attitudes to friendship formation.

2 Encouragement and reinforcement of relations with intimate close friends.

3 Fostering the development of supportive peer groups by placed high value on group identity and group belonging.

Situational conditions that enhance cooperation and those that foster competition will be differentially related to aspects of the environmental climate that may affect loneliness and social competence. Social norms such as an emphasis on the need for every child to have many friends and to be popular may also lead to social difficulties and loneliness. By creating unrealistic expectations about relationships, the environment may increase feelings of social inadequacy and loneliness.

As the target of systemic interventions consists of promoting an environmental change, different change agents have been proposed:

1 Teacher-mediated agents of change.
2 Peer-mediated agents of change.

Teacher-mediated change agents include the teacher's planned praise and reinforcement activities. Peer-mediated change agents include the teacher's activities directed toward the child's classmates, who are themselves trained to create a change. These procedures have been used effectively to increase the social interaction rates of children with and without disabilities (Guevremont, MacMillan, Shawchuck, & Hansen, 1989; McEvoy, Odom, & McConnell, 1992; Kohler, Schwartz, Cross, & Fowler, 1989).

Teacher-mediated intervention

In an example of a teacher-mediated intervention, McEvoy, Odom, and McConnell (1992) found that teachers' prompts and praise for desired social behaviors have an important effect on children's interactions. The teacher can promote and support the type of interactions that may increase and reinforce cooperative task performance and play activities. This approach may focus primarily on the interactions of disabled children in their natural settings, or, as an expression of the systemic approach, may attempt to alter the natural environment through supporting and reinforcing positive social interactions among all of the children, rather than promoting interaction solely within the selected disabled group (Hundert & Houghton, 1992).

Another interesting teacher-mediated program consisted of "affection activities" conducted by teachers, including songs, activities, and prompts for positive social interactions (Brown, Ragland, & Fox, 1988; Twardosz, Nordquist, Simon, & Botkin, 1983). The procedures were called "affection activities" because most prompts for interactions contained expressions of affection (e.g., smiling, hugging), with the aim of increasing interactional activities between the children within the classroom setting.

Peer-mediated intervention

Peer-mediated interventions represent an alternative approach proposing that social change can be engineered through the use of peers as behavior change agents (Guevremont, MacMillan, Shawchuck, & Hansen, 1989). In these interventions, peers are trained to initiate interactions with the target children, such as inviting them to play, reinforcing a desired social activity, and providing social attention. The children's training procedures include role playing in structured situations, monitoring with prompts by adults during social play, and using posters as a reminder and encouragement of the use of the strategy. These peer helpers consist of students in the same school who are taught how to initiate and maintain conversations with target children, as well as how to respond to refusals and how to interact when confronted with negative behaviors.

Such interventions were proven effective for a wide range of children with disabilities and various difficulties (Goldstein & Gallagher, 1992). Several studies have even reported the generalization of positive social behaviors to non-training settings and the maintenance of these gains for up to four months (Guevremont, MacMillan, Shawchuck, & Hansen, 1989; Lancioni, 1982). The introduction of a peer-mediated approach to the remediation of social isolation was found to result in an increase in the children's positive social interactions with both peer helpers and other classmates, to levels comparable to those exhibited by comparison groups. Furman and Bierman (1984) found with preadolescents that a group experience designed to promote involvement with peers increased peer acceptance and self-perceptions of social efficacy.

In evaluating the impact of the training, an important aspect should be considered: In the instruction of certain skills, the effect of the training may be delayed. Bryan and Lee (1990) reported studies in which students failed to show improvement and generalization during the training period but were found to demonstrate such improvement at a follow-up interval 15 weeks later. This is not surprising, especially as related to complex social difficulties such as loneliness; it seems naive to expect long-term social difficulties to change dramatically following short-time interventions. Students' need for intervention and booster sessions may vary in terms of the students' personal temperament and level of understanding of complex environmental information, the length of time required for their training and rehearsal, and the support provided by the environmental climate for the child's attempt to perform his/her newly acquired skills.

Model-based interventions for externalizing maladjustment

As an example of the two approaches for enhancing social competence, intervention research for children with externalizing manifestations of maladjustment will be reported. For reducing disruptive behavior (i.e., aggressive responses), the focus may be placed either on reducing aversive behavior by changing the reinforcement contingencies associated with aversive behaviors, or by building up skilled behaviors (e.g., academic skills or social skills) to substitute or change the disruptive responses within the total repertoire of behavior. Both the systemic approach that aims to achieve an environmental change and the deficit approach that recommends direct training of relevant skills can be found in the intervention research on children with externalizing maladjustment.

Attempts to resocialize aggressive children by eliminating the positive consequences of their maladjusted behavior (Coie & Koeppl, 1990) lead to a systemic approach. In Patterson's (1982) parent-training model, families were trained to eliminate the positive consequences of their children's aggressive behaviors.

The deficit approach featured strategies for coping with anger and teaching self-control to the child with impulsive behavior (Abikoff, 1985; Coie & Koeppl, 1990; Forman, 1980; Lochman, 1985, 1988; Lochman, Bruch, Curry, & Lampron, 1984). Lochman's (1985, 1988) school-based anger-coping training program for aggressive children, within the cognitive-behavioral approach, combined several skill training procedures such as: goal-setting, awareness of body cues related to the arousal of anger, self-statements to inhibit aggressive responses, social problem solving, and stress inoculation. This program, including experimentation with the procedures followed by a short booster training one year later to enhance maintenance and generalization (Lochman, Lampron, Bruch & Curry, 1985), revealed significant effects three years after intervention (Lochman, 1988).

The deficit and the systemic approaches deal with different aspects of aggressive behavior, and each has its advantages and disadvantages. The focus on changing the child's behavior through a parental-training model is based on the belief that the family environmental conditions reinforce and maintain the child's maladaptive behavior. On the other hand, in accordance with a deficit model, only changes in the children's growing self-control skills, problem solving abilities, and coping with anger will enhance the children's resilience.

An alternative approach -- the subtyping model described in Chapter 5, with its emphasis on individualized programming -- adds further justification to the integration of diverse intervention models. The discrimination between proactive and reactive aggression may further illuminate the differential value of each approach for distinct aspects of externalizing maladjustment. For children who use aggression in an instrumental way (i.e., proactive), the contextual approaches may be more appropriate. For children who lose control and burst into anger as a reaction to provocation or stress (i.e., reactive), self-control and skill-training approaches may be more useful.

Integrating the two models: The script intervention

An example of one social skills program that emphasizes the integration of the deficit and systemic models consists of Goldstein and Gallagher's (1992) script intervention program for preschool children. Social scripts are the processes and responses that have been learned and stored in memory, to be used later for the guidance of behaviors and social problem solving. The personal interpretations of social cues based on the child's history of social relations, the memory contents, and the processes used to search memory for a relevant script may increase the likelihood of either aggressive or withdrawn behavior, according to the child's individual style (Huesmann, 1988). This program viewed children's key abilities of developing and sharing scripts for routine events as playing a critical role in social interactions, representing the sharing of common knowledge and expectations within the children's group. The intervention targeted skill deficits by teaching socio-dramatic play skills to preschoolers with language difficulties, in order to enhance the children's verbal interactions. At the same time, the intervention addressed environmental modification through training groups of children in the preschool setting.

Training using a script during the socio-dramatic play involved grouping the children into triads and teaching them scripts comprising different roles and containing behaviors associated with common play scenarios such as going out to eat lunch. The scripts provided a general framework in which groups of children could contribute verbally or nonverbally to a theme. The children each composed and contributed to the script's elaboration, and then they acted it out. The trainer's role was to constantly prompt the children either to stay within their roles or to exchange roles in order to encourage the script's replication with alternative solutions and social problem solving procedures. After the children learned the script and acted it out, they were encouraged to use similar procedures during free play activities to promote generalization (Goldstein & Gallagher, 1992).

The deficit and systemic models of interventions with adults and children as change agents highlighted the value of joining together the different approaches with an eye toward adapting contents and procedures to individuals and system characteristics. The implications for developing interventions to promote children's abilities to cope with their loneliness will be based on these research models and findings for social competence interventions.

Implications for interventions with lonely children

Reviews of the training literature have detailed the richness of approaches and models that differ in intensity and complexity, beginning with the preschool age group and extending through adolescence, for disabled and nondisabled populations alike. These approaches provide a useful axis for efforts to deal effectively with loneliness among children and adolescents. It is already clear that newly acquired coping skills do not translate automatically into more adaptive behavior, requiring the planning of generalization and maintenance as a standard part of intervention programming. Motivational problems and children's willingness to be involved in training should also not be neglected.

Different social skill programs have revealed steps that can be identified within varied perspectives and most approaches (Paris & Oka, 1989):

1. Developing meaningful goals for the target child and his or her peer groups within the contextual climate, as related to the individual's and the group's ways of functioning.

2. Establishing a view of the goals as relevant, thus accounting for the motivation segment, where, for example, the fear of loneliness and the accompanying need to avoid it may constitute a strong motivational factor.

3. Planning the intervention with consideration of both processes and contents, targeting a change in the child and in his/her peer group.

4. Experimenting and demonstrating uses of the strategies to enhance skilled performance.

5. Fostering dialogues between the students and the teacher about strategies, accentuating rule creation and rule following.

6. Planning instruction that promotes generalization and maintenance.

Selection of intervention model

The choice of a model for interventions targeting loneliness among children with disabilities must be closely related to loneliness theory. The conceptualization of loneliness as a multivariate construct related to individual differences and environmental characteristics holds implications for the construction of successful interventions. Interventions should be designed to be concurrently related to sources of loneliness in the individual's current functioning and developmental history, reflecting continuous interactions between environmental and individual goals, and between expectations and attitudes toward solitary activities. Intervention goals should be directed toward changing the child and/or changing the environment in terms of family and school, integrating both the systemic and the skill deficit models to promote satisfying social interactions and to decrease the loneliness experience.

The systemic approach accentuates not only the child who demonstrates interpersonal dissatisfaction and his or her peers, but also the significant adults in the environment. Parents and teachers can create an environment that will promote companionship. They should be encouraged to develop a knowledge base about the social life of their children as early as possible, becoming aware of different developmental aspects such as aggressiveness, shyness, and the identity of their children's friends. Parents can be effective in helping children cope with loneliness by creating opportunities for and encouraging social skills, initiating play activities, and helping children deal with their emotions (Ladd, 1988).

Outside the home, teachers may have an important responsibility not only with regard to creating a learning environment for academic subjects, but also for learning effective and satisfying means of interacting with peers. In a survey of preschool special education teachers, Odom, McConnell, and McEvoy (1992) found that on the average, teachers reported that 75% of the children with disabilities in their classes needed to learn more appropriate and positive ways of interacting with peers. Facing the perceived seriousness of the problem, teachers often feel unprepared to deal with it effectively. Furthermore, in preparing teachers and parents to help children cope effectively with loneliness, the adults' own self-awareness should be developed with regard to their own experiences with loneliness and their attitudes towards solitary activities (Malekoff & Kolodny, 1991). Adults may demonstrate reluctance or difficulty in examining their own feelings of emptiness or isolation, implying the need for support and guidance from intervention planners.

Targeted skill selection

The nature of the social deficiency experienced by lonely children underlies the principles for intervention (Goldstein & Gallagher, 1992) and the different theoretical orientations. Identification of the intervention goals and the deficient skills must be based on individualized assessment and developed within general age-related objectives. Laboratory studies of the social behavior of lonely individuals have also highlighted various aspects of their social skill deficits (Jones, 1982), including negative views of the self and others (Jones, Freemon, & Goswick, 1981), unresponsiveness to others in social interactions (Jones, Hobbs, & Hockenberry, 1982), and inappropriate patterns of self-disclosure (Chelune, Sultan, & Williams, 1980; Solano, Batten, & Parish, 1982). Skill selection should be geared to individual needs, with an emphasis on developmental and systemic considerations.

Procedure selection

Procedures that were found to be effective in social skill training programs, such as modeling, coaching, role playing, and problem solving sequences, should be carefully examined within the loneliness framework. Teacher-mediated and peer-mediated approaches should be applied, in order to initiate change not only within the child who feels lonely and needs training in friendship-making skills, but also in the environment to encourage and promote companionship opportunities (Rizzo, 1988).

A critical question that still remains to be investigated relates to the interactions of children who lack adequate social skills within an environment that highly values and emphasizes these skills. Will children whose disabilities weaken their social skills still require direct training of these skills even within an environment that accentuates social competence, promotes opportunities for social interactions, and appreciates children who develop social interrelations? Interventions seem to be more effective when the targeted children already possess a minimal level of skills and knowledge regarding how to interact within the opportunities provided by the intervention. Assuming that social skills are established via the mutual interaction between the (minimally skilled) child and the (opportunity-providing) environment, the social difficulties of children with disabilities may be even more prominent. For these children, adults' support and intensive skill training must be combined with detailed attention to students' self-reports regarding their social satisfaction and dissatisfaction.

Conclusions

The planning of procedures within interventions for loneliness calls for an awareness of many questions for which the existing social skills research base has not yet provided empirically valid answers. The advantage of complex procedures over simplistic single-dimension interventions (Bierman, Miller, & Stabb, 1987) is not surprising, since any attempt to provide significant answers to long-term difficulties with short-term interventions requires a careful clarification of critical planning questions such as the amount, proportion, and combination of the various procedures. Intervention strategies demand, for instance, careful observations and self-reports concerning the socially penalizing behavior of a child with deficient communication skills, and the identification of functionally equivalent behavior (e.g., asking for access to a play group) to replace the penalized nonaccepted social behavior. Generalization and maintenance will be the ultimate validation of effective interventions, but must also constitute an integral part of the careful planning of procedures. Empirical data has shown that generalization and maintenance of learned skills do not occur automatically and continue to comprise a major difficulty (Hundert & Houghton, 1992), necessitating their inclusion as an inherent component in the training.

Within a systemic model, the loneliness experience can be viewed as one piece of the puzzle of social competence. The systemic model assumes that social relationships are a function of interactions between individuals, the social setting, and values (Vaughn, McIntosh, & Hogan, 1990). Interpersonal relationships are considered both the unit for social understanding and the process for perceiving social order. Social status and peer relations are viewed as part of dynamic, interactive processes in which the child is both influenced by and influences the social processes of others. Through the discernment and formation of a joint view of themselves within their social reality, children's understanding of the self and others is established. Intervention planning should not neglect the subjective perspective on social dissatisfaction, consisting of self-evaluation measures.

Section V
Epilogue: Development, Disabilities, and Loneliness

8 Summary and Future Directions

The impact of the loneliness experience for the adjustment of children with disabilities focused the present discussion on the painful feelings of loneliness and social isolation as revealed in various life contexts: the family environment, school climate, and peer interrelations. My goals in writing this volume were to:

Integrate critical research issues concerning children's connectedness, separateness, and subjective social dissatisfaction as related to disabilities.

Provide a comprehensive working model for understanding the loneliness construct within different environments.

Consolidate psychoanalytic theories of attachment and social learning theories of attribution within the developmental and salutogenic perspectives.

Explore implications from social skill interventional research with the aim of pinpointing effective approaches for changing children's experience of loneliness.

The discussion throughout this volume presented loneliness as a complex construct embodying cognitive, affective, and behavioral aspects. It has been depicted by most people as a distressing and painful experience, but this universal perception of the nature of loneliness does not contradict its unique and subjective meanings for different individuals, reflecting specific and highly personal contents and emotions and their behavioral implications. When two children state that they feel lonely, they are probably referring to different patterns of concerns, beliefs, feelings, and behavioral outcomes. Being lonely may signify a lack of satisfying intimate relations and/or an absence of social identity or belonging to a friendship network. For some children, not being lonely means having one close, loyal friend with whom to share personal and intimate concerns, whereas for other children it means spending most of their free time within a group of peers. In addition to the unique personal meanings of loneliness, the shared aspects of the experience enable different individuals to sense empathy for the loneliness-related pain and unhappiness of others.

The developmental history of children with disabilities is characterized by failures, difficulties, and frustrations, encompassing those encountered in their social world. The inability to satisfy expected needs from one's relational provisions, whether envisioned through Weiss' (1974) social provisions conceptualization or through Josselson's (1992) relatedness dimensions, may be considered as the root of the alienation experience for the child with disabilities. Although parents, teachers, and the disabled youngsters themselves highly value satisfactory social relations and recognize the need to change social interactions, a sense of helplessness is expressed by the youngsters and the significant people in their home and school environments when confronting these goals.

Within the systemic perspective, the self and others can be viewed as one unit that should be studied within a reciprocal paradigm. Feelings of loneliness have been associated with levels of identity and intimacy (Marcoen & Goossens, 1990). The development of aspects of social relations and the sense of self and personal identity all seem to contribute to an explanation of the loneliness experience. For children with and without disabilities, connectedness and separation can be viewed as different components of a process that changes continuously and dynamically within various environments and age stages. Separation from others clarifies the self, leading to greater differentiation and emphasizing firmer personal boundaries, thus enabling more responsiveness to others, because true intimacy is only possible between two separate and independent people (Erickson, 1968). Connectedness to others can be reached when children feel coherent and competent about themselves and are willing to initiate and experiment with interrelations outside of their personal boundaries.

Thus, separations and connections were found to be conceptually interrelated, affecting each other in a reciprocal manner and involving internal and external processes that reflect capacities and disabilities. The internal aspects include multiple components of self-esteem, complex perceptions of others, and various levels of motivation for interrelations. External aspects refer to behaviors that have a clear impact both on the emotional-motivational response and the concept of the self and others.

Loneliness has been conceptualized in this volume as consisting of individual and interpersonal components. Children with disabilities, as a group, were often noted for their lower self-efficacy in various age-related tasks, deficient social skills, and a biased attribution style distinguished by beliefs in the stability, controllability, and globalism of adverse conditions. These personality traits, also found to characterize lonely individuals, were shown to be related to the sense of distress following experiences of alienation and social isolation. Environmental conditions may further promote or limit children's abilities to develop satisfactory human relations. Children's deficiencies in both the connecting and separating processes may predispose them to develop either satisfactory or frustrating interpersonal relations. These predispositions can be understood only through their reciprocal interactions with adults and children within different environmental climates and over time.

The world of the family

Loneliness and social isolation within the family environment is expressed not only by children but also by parents. Confronted with the pain, stress, increased demands, and unwanted life changes introduced by their children's disabilities, parents often reported feeling more lonely. Within the psychoanalytic tradition, it has been accepted that difficulties in early infant-parent relations lead to loneliness at a later developmental stage. The development of attachment relations, separation, and individualization have been considered to be dependent on the reciprocal interrelations between the child and the parents. Recent research on the attachment conceptualization pointed out that stage approaches ignore the dynamic perspective of this construct. It was found that individuals consistently continue negotiating the balance between being close and connected to others and being independent and autonomous or lonely. The general shift of interest within and beyond stage theories toward the more complex dynamics of process theories has been accompanied by a reappraisal of the relations between structure and function, with the contemporary acknowledgement that these dimensions are inseparable. Aspects from the stage theories were integrated into conceptually larger perspectives that respect system dynamics and the fundamental process nature of the experience of development (Mahoney, 1991).

The ecological-systemic approach relates the parent-child difficulties to the family's reactions to the disabling conditions, with a focus on parents' decreased coherence, coping, and affective level and on adverse functioning in the family climate. All of these aspects interact with the child's disabilities and more difficult temperament, leading to higher levels of loneliness both in parents and children. In these families, it was often found that the cohesion and closeness within the family system were decreased, more conflictual relations were reported, and the independence and personal growth of the individual family members were reduced, demonstrating the impact of the children with disabilities on the parents' functioning and thus on the family environment as a whole.

The world of peers

The social learning approach highlighted the nature of peer connectedness outside the family system, illuminating the richness and variability of peer interrelations. The cognitive and emotional difficulties of children with disabilities have often been shown to manifest themselves in prolonged social difficulties. Investigations into the two measures of social relations -- close friendships and belonging to a peer group -- revealed some features of these children's complicated reality. When sociometric measures were utilized, children with disabilities were found in many studies to be represented more within the rejected and neglected groups of children. These children were viewed as demonstrating lower levels of age-appropriate social skills, an attribution bias, and a reputation as rejected individuals, thus further dynamically affecting their social interactions. For many children, rejection by peers was closely related to the experience of loneliness and having a close friendship seemed to mediate loneliness, pinpointing the reciprocal interrelations between the two dimensions within the construct: emotional loneliness and social loneliness.

The study of companionship revealed the full complexity of the process, concentrating on qualitative and quantitative aspects of possessing a good friend. If within the peer world, a good friend is expected to attend to one's major relational needs, then the poorer quality of friendship as reported by individuals with disabilities, and even their desperation due to their unmet expectations for help and support from friendship relations, may clarify their predisposition to social dissatisfaction. Children who remain friendless may be deprived of the very experience with peers that promotes later social development and adjustment. They may be locked into a particularly debilitating social milieu of emotional distress and exclusion from important social resources. However, the heterogeneity of the loneliness experience and the different meanings that children attribute to social relations underscore the importance of attempts to identify subgroups of lonely children.

Subtyping of loneliness and adjustment

Moving from a generalized approach for studying loneliness affords the identification of subgroups to better illustrate the multifaceted nature of the loneliness experience among disabled children. Using Achenbach's (1982) conceptualization of internalizing versus externalizing psychopathology combined with the evaluation of loneliness (Asher, Parkhurst, Hymel, & Williams, 1990), two different subgroups of lonely children and two subgroups of non-lonely children were identified, providing a more differentiated picture.

The behavior of lonely children with disabilities was shown to be classifiable into two subtypes: one group was characterized as withdrawn, introverted, shy, and extremely lonely and isolated; whereas the other lonely group was depicted as aggressive, sometimes hyperactive, and often noted for deficient problem solving, poor social skills, and retaliations of anger and hostility related to attributional bias. Although both of the non-lonely groups of disabled children evidenced good social skills, one non-lonely group demonstrated typical externalizing maladjustment, consisting of aggressive children with age-appropriate leadership abilities and a controversial social status; whereas the other non-lonely group was relatively more adjusted, with introverted tendencies and with disabilities and difficulties focusing in the academic range.

The subtyping model has been found effective for understanding children with learning disabilities and for differentiating between children in two clinical groups: with behavior disorders and with learning disabilities. This approach has much value in explaining maladjustment and loneliness and in guiding individualized intervention planning. For example, training of self-control may be highly valuable for the lonely extroverted group yet harmful for the lonely introverted group, whose behavior can be viewed as overcontrolled and in need of activation and empowerment.

The realization that human behavior is dynamic and individualistic calls for further experimentation in structuring more individualized intervention programs and therapeutic approaches with this model as a guide. Yet, a word of caution is necessary, recognizing that internalizing and externalizing maladjustment features were consistently intermingled in the children, revealing the dynamic forces within relations and conflicts and suggesting that a rigid categorization should be avoided.

Coping and resilience

Individuals not only experience social distress in a unique and subjective manner, but also react to the painful experience of loneliness differently, in their attempts to put an end to the stressful situation. Some feel helpless and sorry for themselves, judging themselves to be ineffective in their coping style. Yet others, even some children with disabilities who experience peer rejection or neglect, reported during interviews that they do not feel lonely very often, implying that are able to demonstrate their resilience and effective coping. The study of different coping strategies among children with disabilities establishes the existence of unique and distinct approaches to stressful situations.

Within the stress and coping paradigm, different children cope with their loneliness using varying levels of approach and avoidance coping. Without ignoring the complex and dynamic patterns of coping strategies, higher levels of passive and avoidance coping with loneliness were evident among the groups of disabled students who were interviewed. In addition, the outcome of coping efforts may be evaluated according to the proportion of solitary versus social activities exhibited in the children's performance repertoire. The study of students with learning disabilities revealed more solitary solutions as coping strategies for reducing loneliness, consisting of solutions where the children were able to become engaged in satisfying activities that can be performed alone. These children preferred to change their inner beliefs, attitudes, and expectations, instead of channelling efforts toward modifying their social relations. Research has suggested that coping should be treated as a combined pattern of different activities including solitary and group efforts. Only careful and detailed investigations into the private world of the loneliness experience, as viewed by different children, may result in the design of effective, individualized interventions.

We should not ignore the interesting fact that in several interview studies, about one-quarter of the samples refused to answer the questions relating to how they behaved at times when they felt lonely. These children were reluctant to share their private experience and to disclose their intimate hurts. Although we do not have information on their experiences, children who attempt to avoid dealing with their sense of loneliness may be considered at risk, requiring special attention in the planning of interventions.

Empowering the lonely child

Within a salutogenic orientation (Antonovsky, 1987) that attempts to identify factors promoting activities located at the healthy end of the continuum, that aim to foster socialization or decrease loneliness without focusing on the causes or roots of distress, the empowerment approach has been employed. Three basic assumptions underlie the empowerment approach to intervention planning (Margalit, 1990a):

1 *Competence.* Children possess the capacity for coping with their loneliness or the potential to become competent.

2 *Enabling experience.* The systemic climate creates opportunities for competencies to be displayed.

3 *Sense of control.* Children's attributions and beliefs reflect their sense of control over behavioral changes.

Empowerment has often been viewed as the process that facilitates the individual's identification and recognition of needs and the ability to use existing personal competencies in order to obtain resources to meet these needs. Within this approach, the identification of the sources of an individual's loneliness comprises the precondition for intervention programming.

The social difficulties of lonely children may reflect one or a combination of the following three factors:

1 *A knowledge deficit.* The child has not acquired the appropriate knowledge and skills needed at that age level to develop satisfactory social relations.

2 *A performance defect.* The child has not captured the ability to translate social skills and knowledge into effective behavior that enhances satisfying companionship relations.

3 *A role affiliation.* The child has adopted the characteristics and behaviors typical of lonely children, developing a reputation as an isolated individual and beliefs as to how a lonely child should behave.

Students with disabilities, whose loneliness is closely related to deficient social skills and who failed to acquire age-related social abilities, need social skill instruction. In the future, detailed investigations will be needed to clarify the deficient information processes that may comprise the roots of these skill deficits.

Students whose disabilities are expressed in performance difficulties, originating in ineffective translations of existing social knowledge, may need step-by-step guidance for successful performance of their social knowledge. Training and experimenting within sheltered and naturalistic environments will provide them with the needed opportunities for direct experiences to foster the achievement of skilled and fluent performance.

The role affiliation factor is often neglected yet is especially valuable in empowering interventions and is closely related to research on the characteristics of lonely individuals. Self-cognitions and personal role definitions may have a strong impact on social behaviors. The development of an identity of the self as a lonely or coherent individual may affect behavior directly and indirectly. Lonely children's behaviors reflect their own perceived self-definitions and identifications and may include components stemming from their expectations that other children will reject or ignore them. Their behaviors may already incorporate reactions to these expectations, in terms of withdrawal or disruptiveness, thus perpetuating the cycle of peer rejection. Indirectly, these children also have less motivation to learn new social skills or to experiment with them, contributing to a growth in their secondary developmental delay in social competence.

Personal and social change following successful interventions rely extensively on different methods of empowerment (Bandura, 1988) such as providing individuals with knowledge, skills, and resilient self-beliefs of efficacy to alter aspects of their lives over which they have control. Personal beliefs and perceived self-efficacy about one's capabilities to organize and implement the actions necessary for attaining designated levels of performance in different areas have been found important in mediating behavioral change (Schunk, Hanson, & Cox, 1987). Judgements of personal efficacy affect the individual's choice of activities and selection of environments (Ozer & Bandura, 1990). Individuals tend to avoid activities and situations they believe will exceed their coping capabilities, but they readily undertake activities and select and become involved in social environments that they judge themselves capable of handling (Bandura, 1989). On the other hand, personal expectations for success have been viewed as leading to greater persistence of efforts and motivation. The sources of self-motivation rely on two main aspects of the intervening processes: goal setting and self-evaluation. This form of self-motivation, which operates largely through internal comparison processes, requires personal standards against which to evaluate ongoing performance (Bandura & Schunk, 1981).

Personal goals do not automatically activate the evaluative process that affects an individual's social behavior. Various properties of these goals, such as their levels of specialty and the existence of attainable subgoals, help to provide a clearer standard of adequacy, thereby initiating greater motivation. Children who set themselves attainable subgoals were shown to progress more rapidly in their self-directed learning, achieve better mastery of learned skills, heighten their perceived self-efficacy, and increase their interest in activities leading to the achievement of the desired goal (Bandura & Schunk, 1981).

To reach the desired change in self-efficacy, modeling has been found valuable, in view of the fact that it implicitly conveys to the observers that they are capable of performing the modeled operation. The advantages of peer modeling over teacher modeling were demonstrated in Schunk and Hanson's (1985) study, suggesting that children's perceived similarity to models' competence levels may further influence their self-efficacy. The individualistic approaches to empowerment interventions within a comprehensive model of children's transactional interrelations require detailed assessment of the individual child's functioning levels, specific self-beliefs in the targeted interpersonal areas of functioning, and global self-perceptions in terms of the sense of coherence conceptualization. Human change is integrally related to self-system issues, and human relatedness plays an important role in self-system development (Mahoney, 1991).

Transactional relations

The empowerment process can be fully understood only within the context of the interpersonal behavior model. Vitkus and Horowitz (1987) suggested a contemporary version of an interpersonal model of personality that may be useful in discerning the transactional relations within the development of loneliness. The model assumes that the study of interpersonal behaviors can be organized along two orthogonal dimensions: control (from dominance to submissiveness) and affiliation (from hostility to companionship).

Children reciprocally affect each other through their interactions, and their behaviors are interdependent. The behaviors of one child tend to elicit particular classes of reactions that may be characterized as reciprocal with respect to the control dimension or may be depicted as corresponding with respect to the affiliation dimension. For example, if one child, in a hostile, dominant reaction, rejects the request of a disabled child to join the group of children who are playing together, then the rejected child is apt to become defensive, expressing either hostile submissiveness or withdrawn submissiveness.

The child with disabilities who expresses distress and asks for help (i.e., submissive friendliness) may enlist the willingness of a peer to support and help (i.e., dominant friendliness) or may meet with a peer who reacts angrily and negatively (i.e., dominant hostility). Children with disabilities often behave in ways that express submissiveness, inviting other children to react to them in dominating patterns -- either friendly or hostile -- and thus reaffirming and sustaining their role expectations and self-definitions. These dominating responses elicit even further submissive reactions from the lonely child, thereby perpetuating their lonely patterns of behavior and their feelings of helplessness and social inadequacy. When children accept a basically submissive and passive role, their social deficits in both knowledge and performance will be accentuated. This conceptualization emphasized the need for further study of the social interactions with peers who are disabled and nondisabled.

Only well-designed intervention programs have the potential for placing these children into a relatively active role that can facilitate effective coping, enhance their skill learning through modeling and training, and lead to increased resilience and adjustment. In order to design effective and empowering interventions, these self-perpetuating interaction sequences must first be studied in detail and second be examined for the means and timing to interrupt the maladjusted interpersonal role cycle. Creating tasks and changing performance and self-evaluation may be important components in empowering interventions. The importance of the instruction and training of social skills and fluent performance should not be overlooked; however, it should be recognized that lonely individuals who adopt a passive role are less likely to benefit from skill training. If these children approach social situations with anxiety and beliefs of their inadequacy, their submissive behavior will elicit more dominant reactions from other children. Future research is needed to experiment with various procedures to activate the lonely inactive child.

Diversity in social functioning

Loneliness may lead to anxiety and avoidance. It has been extremely valuable to reveal that children, even extremely lonely ones, expressed during their interviews a strong motivation to have friends and not to stay alone. The motivations and expectations related to having social relations are important in designing interventions. The interviewing process revealed that several children believed in their abilities to control social situations and were creative in suggesting different solutions for coping. Other children revealed a coping difficulty that was accompanied by high levels of subjective distress and anxiety. The role of the perceived self-efficacy in controlling negative cognitions and thoughts takes on increased significance in relation to these children's growing anxiety. Activating the passive and withdrawn child calls for continuous attempts and experimentation within the empowering construct.

Active problem solving has been found to be related to well-being and positive affect, and a transactional process was identified between avoidance coping and personal distress. In Ebata and Moos' (1991) study, distressed adolescents demonstrated more involvement in avoidance coping, and those adolescents who were engaged in such coping were found to adjust more poorly when confronted with life stressors. These passive tendencies were shown to be interrelated with stress and maladjustment throughout extensive research (Ebata & Moos, 1991).

Children may be considered social beings who certainly need interactions with others, both with adults and peers, yet considerable variation exists in the depth and frequency of the relationships that individuals need and establish with one another. Human diversity has also been expressed by the varying levels of involvement in different areas of solitary and companionable interest and by the heterogeneous nature of interpersonal relationships. Children's activities are geared toward the impersonal as well as toward the personal (Storr, 1988). The developmental course, inherited gifts and capacities, temperamental differences and disabilities, and a host of other factors may influence whether individuals turn predominantly toward others or toward solitude.

The capacity to be alone is considered a valuable resource that facilitates learning, thinking, coming to terms with change, and the maintenance of contact with the inner world of imagination and dreams. Adaptation to stressful situations is closely related to the development of imagination and the inner world that generates attitudes and beliefs about the self and the outer world. It still remains to be investigated whether the loneliness of children with disabilities can be viewed as an additional manifestation of their maturational delay, specifically of a delay in their ability to stay alone and become involved in satisfactory interests.

Interventions for lonely children can be considered effective only if they lead to the experience of change in this private reality -- in meanings, emotions, behaviors, and relations (Mahoney, 1991). The empowering models center efforts toward promoting changes in the processes and outcomes that are directed at the children's experiences of themselves as related to others, both peers and adults. Within the intervention research database, the value of social skill training was not ignored, yet the focus of loneliness interventions seems to be moving toward enhancing a more global change, with the social skills and problem solving procedures providing only a partial answer for the social distress. These interventions should emphasize the activation of the individual to search for individualistic answers to social needs and goals and should foster the ability both to develop meaningful connections and to develop areas of interest for enjoyable solitary activities.

Among the psychological needs of children, three interrelated areas may be underscored as fundamental for academic learning and social growth (Ryan & Powelson, 1991): autonomy, relatedness, and competence.

1 *Autonomy.* The term autonomy refers to regulating one's own behavior, experiences, and personal boundaries. Self-determination and self-regulations are related concepts in the definition of the autonomy striving.

2 *Relatedness.* The term relatedness refers to regulating the distance between oneself and others. Children's relations with peers and adults may be characterized either as close or as superficial contacts and may be shaped in order to fulfill the supportive function of provider or else to play the role of the receiver who is supported by the different provisions.

3 *Competence.* Competence concerns the sense of accomplishment and effectiveness under conditions of

> challenge. The sense of competence may mediate autonomy striving and the need for the establishment of relatedness.

In autonomous experiences the locus of causality lies within the self, emphasizing the independent self as contrasted with the concept of relatedness that concerns emotional and personal relations. Personal competence may serve as a mediating force between the dynamically interrelating needs of independence/dependence and of relatedness/isolation. In schools where children are supported in their attempt to reach autonomy and to experience competence, without denying their need to feel the relatedness to others available only through social interrelations, the children can be expected to reveal more involvement in their learning.

However, children with disabilities are seldom able to achieve levels of competence in many age-related tasks, further affecting their loneliness and dependence. Children who have disabilities face many situations and tasks that they cannot perform, thus feeling incompetent and demonstrating lower self-esteem. Systemic interventions may do well to target those contexts and tasks where students can experience autonomy and competence yet also feel connected to the performing group. It appears that the interpersonal dimensions of autonomy, support, and relatedness represent important forces in the affective and cognitive outcomes of schooling. The recognition of the centrality of the interpersonal atmosphere in fostering learning and growth may be valuable in directing prevention efforts.

9 Issues for Further Exploration

In the course of writing this volume, I have had the opportunity to enter into many discussions with colleagues in Israel and abroad as well as with students at Tel Aviv University and psychologists and special education teachers. These productive exchanges elicited a number of meaningful issues that were not crucial to the development of the argument in this book. Yet if my aim is to convey the full richness of the loneliness conceptualization as related to children with disabilities, it seems appropriate to add here some suggestions for reflection and exploration.

I will first discuss the salutogenic question in the context of loneliness research. Next, to further clarify the recommended directions for intervention planning, the issue of the psychologist-educator-parent role interface will be raised. The third topic will consist of an examination of future research questions.

Sense of coherence and loneliness

My primary goal has been to suggest a working conceptual system within the salutogenic model for empowering children with disabilities, through a focus on their loneliness and social dissatisfaction experience. Discussing loneliness may seem appropriate within the pathogenic orientation, but rather paradoxical and controversial when the accent is on resilience and empowerment. However, within Antonovsky's (1987) salutogenic approach, the loneliness discussion as presented in this volume leads first of all to the realization of the heterogeneity of human experience, and secondly to viewing the loneliness-companionship construct not as a dichotomy between lonely and not lonely children, but rather as a continuum.

It has been a professional challenge to investigate the position of children with disabling conditions along this continuum, while taking into consideration the dynamically changing experiences of connectedness and loneliness among various people who have individual needs at different periods of time and within distinct environmental climates. I believe that the clarification of individualized effective coping strategies, even among disabled children, will help mobilize these individuals according to their unique personal needs, goals, and subjective preferences.

During the last three years I met with teachers, counselors, parents, and university students to discuss the loneliness experience in the special education system. My goals were to clarify the sources and expressions of the alienation feelings of children with disabilities. My amazement grew in response to the strong emotional reactions and spontaneous self-references I received, as I went from one meeting to another. These adults expressed their feelings of being emotionally moved by children's loneliness and shared their personal memories from their own lonely experiences of childhood. They felt distressed by and uncomfortable with children's loneliness and expressed a readiness to become involved and invest great efforts and a vast amount of time toward enhancing social growth, if the appropriate training would be provided.

I was appreciative of their excitement and eagerness to help the children enter into age-appropriate social relations. Yet, although these professionals fully recognized their own needs for solitude, they did not attribute sufficient importance to strengthening the ability of children with disabilities to develop the capacity to stay alone.

Before introducing changes in the children's connectedness and loneliness experience, their experience of solitude must be studied within different contextual conditions. Time spent alone may be used for creative activities, enjoyable interests, or serious investment in an area of great personal value. Along the continuum of being with others and staying alone, different levels of self-satisfaction and self-coherence may be experienced. Thus, assessment and intervention should be conceptualized within the salutogenic model, aiming at enhancing the sense of coherence of disabled children through a comprehensive understanding of their loneliness and connectedness, as they continuously change and develop at different ages.

Change and change agents

The goals of loneliness interventions should be to promote changes within relatively stable domains such as social status and interaction patterns and across a variety of social situations. Three basic assumptions on which all psychological and educational interventions rest have been suggested by Mahoney (1991):

1 Humans can change, yet there are constraints on human plasticity.

2 Human beings can help others to change, but they can also with the best intentions hinder such changes.

3 Some forms of helping are more effective than others in facilitating change.

Children with disabilities can change, and individuals in their environments can help them in the changing process. Parents, peers, and teachers may create supportive environments to foster companionship relations and also may promote more direct changes in social interactions through instruction, modeling, coaching, and therapy. The optimal system for promoting changes in children's functioning is the one that provides a secure, developmentally flexible, and fundamentally caring environment.

In the specialized realm of creating a change through intervention and therapy, the process has been considered significantly affected by the personal characteristics of the therapist and teacher, especially in terms of the interventional skills and the quality of relations he or she can co-create with the children in need. Psychologists and mental health professionals who have received training in various therapeutic procedures and interventions that aim to modify human relations are notable in their feelings of being more skilled in this area. However, in order to initiate a systemic change, all the participants -- parents, children, and teachers -- must actively participate as agents of change. Yet teachers and parents alike often feel reluctant to become involved in initiating changes within social-emotional spheres.

The role of the mental health expert will be different in various contexts and time periods. Individual therapists attempt to provide the lonely child with an experience of confidence in human relations and to enhance the development of a robust self-identity through the creation of a therapeutic relationship. Another professional may target context engineering, where different individuals are trained within the environment as a whole, in an attempt to change its social climate, provide more opportunities for cooperation and companionship, increase the supportiveness and warmth of the environment, and at the same time map out the instruction of the needed skills.

This complex approach recommending an interface of the professional, parent, and educator must simultaneously attend to the multiple factors that predict social relations and the sense of loneliness. For instance, interventions with a focus on stable environments may need to incorporate contextual components such as the inclusion of peers as change agents. Teachers, parents, and peers can learn to be effective change agents in helping children with disabilities to cope more effectively with their loneliness experience. A systemic approach could help to clarify the full power and interplay between developmental processes of social relations in the different environments. In this way, school, family, and peer group settings can be viewed as interrelated systems whose impacts on the child are linked together, shaping the student's growth and performance.

Combined processes that promote changes in the child, and at the same time target changes in the system and in significant individuals in the environment to support the social change in the child, may decrease loneliness. Such a systemic perspective may also have implications for destabilizing the consistent carry-over effect of social status on different social situations (Luftig, 1987). Yet, intervention planning for long-term difficulties such as loneliness among children with disabilities should recollect Mahoney's (1991) suggestion that significant changes rarely occur easily or rapidly.

Future research directions

The study of loneliness, disabilities, and interventions is at its initial stages. The clarification of the loneliness construct for this special population continues to require intensive investigation. However, several research questions seem more critical at the present level of study. The heterogeneity revealed through research in the loneliness experience among children with and without disabilities should be further explored, calling for in-depth investigations on the subjective experience, using varied procedures. Research directed at identifying predictors of loneliness and of children's resilience, attending to individual and systemic differences, will be valuable in elucidating the construct.

The consistency of the loneliness experience is another critical question that should not be ignored. Everybody feels lonely from time to time. Yet some children stay lonely for longer periods, feeling more desperate. Research into temporary changes and environmental conditions as they interact with individual competencies and disabilities may advance our working model of how the experience develops.

When children say that they are lonely, they mean different things. The investigation of the various aspects and meanings of loneliness and companionship among children with disabilities, as related to stressful social events in their home and school systems, may add to theoretical understanding and contribute toward effective intervention planning. Research using controlled individualistic and systemic interventions is also critical for introducing significant changes.

An attempt has been made to clarify the meaning of loneliness as a subjective experience among children with disabilities, through the presentation of a model and of directions for research and intervention. It should be remembered that the goals for change and intervention can help these youngsters, yet have their own innate constraints. Disabilities affect the children's competencies, even within the most supportive environment. Only individualistic, dynamic, and complex considerations may promise these children and their families a better future with effective routes toward attaining greater satisfaction from themselves as unique and autonomous individuals and from their social interrelations.

References

Abikoff, H. (1985). Efficacy of cognitive training interventions in hyperactive children: A critical review. *Clinical Psychological Review, 5,* 479-512.

Abramson, L. Y., Seligman, M. E. P., & Teasdale, J. (1978). Learned helplessness in humans: Critique and reformulation. *Journal of Abnormal Psychology, 87,* 49-74.

Achenbach, T. M. (1982). *Developmental psychopathology* (2nd ed.). New York: Wiley.

Achenbach, T. M., & Edelbrock, C. (1983). *Manual for the child behavior checklist and revised child behavior profile.* University of Vermont: Department of Psychiatry.

Ainsworth, M. D. (1990). Some considerations regarding theory and assessment relevant to attachments beyond infancy. In M. T. Greenberg, D. Cicchetti, & E. M. Cummings (Eds.), *Attachment in preschool years* (pp. 463-488). Chicago: University of Chicago Press.

Altman, I. (1975). *The environment and social behavior: Privacy, personal space, crowding.* Monterey, CA: Brools-Cole.

Anderson, C. A., & Arnoult, L. H. (1985). Attributional style and everyday problems in living: Depression, loneliness and shyness. *Social Cognition, 3,* 16-35.

Anderson, C. A., & Riger, A. L. (1991). A controllability attributional model of problems in living: Dimensional and situational interactions in the prediction of depression and loneliness. *Social Cognition, 9,* 149-181.

Andersson, L. (1985). Loneliness, birth order and social loss among a group of elderly women. *Journal of Psychosomatic Research, 29,* 33-42.

Andersson, L. (1986). A model of estrangement - including a theoretical understanding of loneliness. *Psychological Reports, 58,* 689-695.

Andersson, L. (1990). Narcissism and loneliness. *Aging and Human Development, 30,* 81-94.

Andersson, L., Mullins, L. C., & Johnson, D. P. (1987). Parental intrusion versus social isolation: A dichotomous view of the sources of loneliness. In M. Hojat, & R. Crandall (Eds.),

Loneliness: Theory, research and applications [Special Issue]. *Journal of Social Behavior and Personality, 2,* 125-134.

Andrasik, F., & Matson, J. L. (1985). Social skills training for the mentally retarded. In L. L'Abate (Ed.), *Handbook of social skill training and research* (pp. 418-453). New York: Wiley.

Antonovsky, A. (1979). *Health, stress and coping.* San Francisco: Jossey-Bass.

Antonovsky, A. (1987). *Unraveling the mystery of health.* San Francisco: Jossey-Bass.

Antonovsky, A., & Sourani, T. (1988). Family sense of coherence and family adaptation. *Journal of Marriage and the Family, 50,* 79-92.

Asher, S. R. (1983). Social competence and peer status: Recent advances and future directions. *Child Development, 54,* 1427-1434.

Asher, S. R., Hymel, S., & Renshaw, P. D. (1984). Loneliness in children. *Child Development, 55,* 1456-1464.

Asher, S. R., Parkhurst, J. T., Hymel, S., & Williams, G. A. (1990). Peer rejection and loneliness in childhood. In S. R. Asher, & J. D. Coie (Eds.), *Peer rejection in childhood* (pp. 253-273). Cambridge, England: University Press.

Asher, S. R., & Renshaw, P. D. (1981). Children without friends: Social knowledge and social skills. In S. R. Asher, & J. M. Gottman (Eds.), *The development of children's friendships* (pp. 273-296). New York: Cambridge University Press.

Asher, S. R., & Wheeler, V. A. (1985). Children's loneliness: A comparison of rejected and neglected peer status. *Journal of Consulting and Clinical Psychology, 53,* 500-505.

Avison, W. R., & Turner, R. J. (1988). Stressful life events and depressive symptoms: Disaggregating the effects of acute stressors and chronic strains. *Journal of Health and Social Behavior, 29,* 253-264.

Avrahami, J. (1992). *Social competence and loneliness among two groups of students with mild mental retardation.* Unpublished Master's thesis, Tel Aviv University.

Bandura, A. (1977). *Social learning theory.* Englewood Cliffs, NJ: Prentice-Hall.

Bandura, A. (1986). *Social foundations of thought and action: A social cognitive theory.* Englewood Cliffs, NJ: Prentice-Hall.

Bandura, A. (1988). Self-efficacy conception of anxiety. *Anxiety Research, 1,* 77-98.

Bandura, A. (1989). Regulation of cognitive processes through perceived self-efficacy. *Developmental Psychology, 255,* 729-735.

Bandura, A., & Schunk, D. H. (1981). Cultivating competence, self-efficacy and intrinsic interest through proximal self-motivation. *Journal of Personality and Social Psychology, 41,* 586-598.

Bandura, A., & Wood, R. (1989). Effects of perceived controllability and performance standards on self-regulation of complex decision making. *Journal of Personality and Social Psychology, 56,* 805-814.

Bear, G. G., Clever, A., & Proctor, W. A. (1991). Self-perceptions of nonhandicapped children and children with learning disabilities. *Journal of Special Education, 24,* 409-426.

Bell, R. A. (1991). Gender, friendship network density, and loneliness. *Journal of Social Behavior and Personality, 6,* 45-56.

Berndt, T. J. (1981). The effects of friendship on prosocial intentions and behavior. *Child Development, 52,* 636-643.

Berndt, T. J. (1990, April). *Relations of friendships and peer acceptance to adolescents' self-evaluation.* Paper presented at the annual American Educational Research Association conference, Boston.

Bierman, K. L. (1986a). Process of change during social skills training with preadolescents and its relation to treatment outcome. *Child Development, 57,* 230-240.

Bierman, K. L. (1986b). The relation between social aggression and peer rejection in middle childhood. In R. J. Prinz (Ed.), *Advances in behavioral assessment of children and families* (Vol. 2, pp. 151-178). New York: JAI Press.

Bierman, K. L., Miller, C. L., & Stabb, S. D. (1987). Improving the social behavior and peer acceptance of rejected boys: Effects of social skill training with instructions and prohibitions. *Journal of Consulting and Clinical Psychology, 55,* 194-200.

Billings, A. G., & Moos, R. H. (1981). The role of coping responses and social resources in attenuating the stress of life events. *Journal of Behavioral Medicine, 4,* 139-157.

Blacher, J., Nihira, K., & Meyers, C. E. (1987). Characteristics of home environment of families with mentally retarded children: Comparison across levels of retardation. *American Journal of Mental Deficiency, 91,* 313-320.

Bolea, A. S. (1986). Treating loneliness in children. *Psychotherapy Patient, 2,* 15-27.

Borkowski, J. G., Day, J. D., Saenz, D., Dietmeyer, D., Estrada, T. M., & Groteluschen, A. (1992). Expanding the boundaries of cognitive interventions. In Y. L. Wong (Ed.), *Contemporary intervention research in learning disabilities: An international perspective* (pp. 1-21). New York: Springer-Verlag.

Bowlby, J. (1973). *Attachment and loss: Separation* (Vol. 2). New York: Basic Books.

Bowlby, J. (1988). *A secure base.* New York: Basic Books.

Boyce, G. C., Behl, D., Mortensen, L., & Akers, J. (1991). Child characteristics, family demographics and family processes: Their effects on the stress experienced by families of children with disabilities. *Counseling Psychology Quarterly, 4,* 273-288.

Breen, M. J., & Barkley, R. A. (1988). Child psychopathology and parenting stress in girls and boys having attention deficit disorder with hyperactivity. *Journal of Pediatric Psychology, 13,* 265-280.

Breiner, J., & Young, D. L. (1985). Social interaction: A comparison of mothers with noncompliant, nondelayed and developmentally delayed children. *Child & Family Behavior Therapy, 7,* 1-7.

Brennan, T. (1982). Loneliness at adolescence. In L. A. Peplau, & D. Perlman (Eds.), *Loneliness: A sourcebook of current theory, research and therapy* (pp. 269-290). New York: Wiley.

Bristol, M. M., Gallagher, J. J., & Schopler, E. (1988). Mothers and fathers of young developmentally disabled and nondisabled boys: Adaptation and spousal support. *Developmental Psychology, 24,* 441-451.

Bronfenbrener, U. (1979). *The ecology of human development: Experiments by nature and design.* Cambridge, MA: Harvard University Press.

Bronfenbrener, U. (1986). Ecology of the family as a context for human development: Research perspectives. *Developmental Psychology, 22,* 723-742.

Brown, W. H., Ragland, E. U., & Fox, J. J. (1988). Effects of group socialization procedures on the social interactions of preschool children. *Research in Developmental Disabilities, 9,* 359-376.

Bruininks, V. L. (1978). Actual and perceived peer status of learning disabled students in mainstreamed programs. *Journal of Special Education, 12,* 51-58.

Bryan, T. H. (1974). Peer popularity of learning disabled children. *Journal of Learning Disabilities, 7,* 621-625.

Bryan, T. H., & Bryan, J. H. (1978). Social interactions of learning disabled children. *Learning Disabilities Quarterly, 1,* 33-38.

Bryan, T. H., & Lee, J. (1990). Social skills training with learning disabled children and adolescents: The state of art. In T. E. Scruggs, & B. Y. L. Wong (Eds.), *Intervention research in learning disabilities* (pp. 263-278). New York: Springer-Verlag.

Bryan, T. H., Pearl, R., & Fallon, P. (1989). Conformity to peer pressure by students with learning disabilities: A replication. *Journal of Learning Disabilities, 22,* 458-459.

Burden, R., & Thomas, D. (1986). A further perspective on parental reaction to handicap. *Exceptional Child, 33,* 140-145.

Burke, P. J., & McDonnell, J. H. (1992). Enthusiastic and growing. In R. Fessler, & J. C. Christensen (Eds.), *The teacher career cycle* (pp. 119-151). Boston: Allyn & Bacon.

Burns, M. O., & Seligman, M. E. P. (1989). Explanatory style across the lifespan: Evidence for stability over 52 years. *Journal of Personality and Social Psychology, 56,* 471-477.

Cairns, R. B., & Cairns, B. D. (1984). Predicting aggressive patterns in girls and boys: A developmental study. *Aggressive Behavior, 10,* 227-242.

Cantrell, V. L., & Prinz, R. J. (1985). Multiple perspectives of rejected, neglected and accepted children: Relations between sociometric status and behavioral characteristics. *Journal of Consulting and Clinical Psychology, 53,* 884-889.

Carver, C. S., Scheier, M. F., & Weintraub, J. K. (1989). Assessing coping strategies: A theoretically based approach. *Journal of Personality and Social Psychology, 56,* 267-283.

Cassidy, J., & Asher, S. R. (1992). Loneliness and peer relations in young children. *Child Development, 63,* 350-365.

Cassidy, J., Parke, R. D., Butkovsky, L., & Braungart, J. M. (1992). Family-peer connections: The role of emotional expressiveness within the family and children's understanding of emotions. *Child Development, 63,* 603-618.

Cheek, J. M., & Busch, C. M. (1981). The influence of shyness on loneliness in a new situation. *Personality and Social Psychology Bulletin, 7,* 572-577.

Chelune, G. J., Sultan, F. E., & Williams, C. L. (1980). Loneliness, self-disclosure and interpersonal effectiveness. *Journal of Consulting Psychology, 27,* 462-468.

Cicchetti, D., Cummings, E. M., Greenberg, M. T., & Marvin, R. S. (1990). An organizational perspective on attachment beyond infancy: Implications for theory, measurement and research. In M. T. Greenberg, D. Cicchetti, & E. M. Cummings (Eds.), *Attachment in preschool years* (pp. 3-49). Chicago: University of Chicago Press.

Cillessen, A. H. N., Van Lieshout, C. F. M., & Haselager, G. J. T. (1992, August). *Children's problems caused by consistent rejection in early elementary school.* Paper presented at the annual American Psychological Association convention, Washington, DC.

Clark, L. A., & Watson, D. (1988). Mood and the mundane: Relations between daily life events and self-reported mood. *Journal of Personality and Social Psychology, 54,* 296-308.

Clegg, J. A., & Standen, P. J. (1991). Friendship among adults who have developmental disabilities. *American Journal of Mental Retardation, 95,* 663-671.

Cohen, D. S., & Wills, T. A. (1985). Stress, social support, and the buffering hypothesis. *Psychological Bulletin, 98,* 310-357.

Coie, J. D. (1985). Fitting social skills intervention to the target group. In B. H. Schneider, K. H. Rubin, & J. E. Ledingham (Eds.), *Peer relationships and social skills in childhood: Issues in assessment and training* (pp.141-150). New York: Springer-Verlag.

Coie, J. D. (1990). Toward a theory of peer rejection. In S. R. Asher, & J. D. Coie (Eds.), *Peer rejection in childhood* (pp. 365-401). Cambridge, England: University Press.

Coie, J. D., & Dodge, K. A. (1983). Continuities and changes in children's social status: A five-year longitudinal study. *Merrill-Palmer Quarterly, 29,* 261-282.

Coie, J. D., Dodge, K. A., & Coppotelli, H. (1982). Dimensions and types of social status: A cross-age perspective. *Developmental Psychology, 18,* 557-570.

Coie, J. D., Dodge, K. A., & Kupersmidt, J. B. (1990). Peer group behavior and social status. In S. R. Asher, & J. D. Coie (Eds.), *Peer rejection in childhood* (pp. 17-59). Cambridge, England: University Press.

Coie, J. D., & Koeppl, G. K. (1990). Adapting intervention to the problems of aggressive and disruptive rejected children. In S. R. Asher, & J. D. Coie (Eds.), *Peer rejection in childhood* (pp. 309-337). Cambridge, England: University Press.

Coie, J. D., & Kupersmidt, J. A. (1983). A behavioral analysis of emerging social status in boys' groups. *Child Development, 54,* 1400-1416.

Coyne, J. C., & Lazarus, R. S. (1981). Cognitive style, stress perception and coping. In I. L. Kutash, & L. B. Schlesinger (Eds.), *Handbook on stress and anxiety* (pp. 144-158). San Francisco: Jossey-Bass.

Cramer, P., & Skidd, J. E. (1992). Correlates of self-worth in preschoolers: The role of gender-stereotyped styles of behavior. *Sex Roles, 26,* 369-390.

Crnic, K. A., Friedrich, W. N., & Greenberg, M. T. (1983). Adaptation of families with mentally retarded children: A model of stress, coping, and family ecology. *American Journal of Mental Deficiency, 88,* 125-138.

Crnic, K. A., Greenberg, M. T., Ragozin, A., Robinson, N., & Basham, R. (1983). Effects of stress and social support on mothers of premature and full-term infants. *Child Development, 54,* 209-217.

Csikszentmihalyi, M., & Larson, R. (1984). *Being adolescent.* New York: Basic Books.

Cummings, E. M. (1990). Classification of attachment on a continuum of the felt security: Illustrations from the study of depressed parents. In M. T. Greenberg, D. Cicchetti, & E. M. Cummings (Eds.), *Attachment in preschool years* (pp. 311-338). Chicago: University of Chicago Press.

Cummings, E. M., & Cicchetti, D. (1990). Toward a transactional model of relations between attachment and depression. In M. T. Greenberg, D. Cicchetti, & E. M. Cummings (Eds.), *Attachment in preschool years* (pp. 339-372). Chicago: University of Chicago Press.

Cummings, E. M., Iannotti, R. J., & Zahn-Waxler, C. (1985). Influence of conflict between adults on the emotion and aggression of young children. *Developmental Psychology, 21,* 495-507.

Cummings, E. M., Zahn-Waxler, C., & Radke-Yarrow, M. (1981). Young children's responses to expressions of anger and affection by others in the family. *Child Development, 52,* 1274-1282.

Darling, R. B. (1988). Parental entrepreneurship: A consumerist response to professional dominance. *Journal of Social Issues, 44,* 141-158.

Davis, M. H., & Franzoi, S. L. (1986). Adolescent loneliness, self-disclosure, and private self-consciousness: A longitudinal investigation. *Journal of Personality and Social Psychology, 51*, 595-608.

Day, D. M., Bream, L. A., & Pal, A. (1992). Proactive and reactive aggression: An analysis of subtypes based on teacher perception. *Journal of Clinical Child Psychology, 21*, 210-217.

Deal, A. G., Trivette, C. M., & Dunst, C. J. (1988). Family functioning style. In C. J. Dunst, C. M. Trivette, & A. G. Deal (Eds.), *Enabling and empowering families: Principles and guidelines for practice* (pp. 179-184). Cambridge, MA: Brookline.

Denham, S. A. (1986). Social cognition, prosocial behavior and emotion in preschoolers: Contextual validation. *Child Development, 57*, 194-201.

Denham, S. A. (1989). Maternal affect and toddlers' social-emotional competence. *American Journal of Orthopsychiatry, 59*, 368-376.

Denham, S. A., McKinley, M., Couchoud, E. A., & Holt, R. (1990). Emotional and behavioral predictors of preschool peer ratings. *Child Development, 61*, 1145-1152.

Denham, S. A., Zahn-Waxler, C., Cummings, E. M., & Iannotti, R. J. (1991). Social competence in young children's peer relations: Patterns of development and change. *Child Psychiatry and Human Development, 22*, 29-44.

Derlega, V. J., & Margulis, S. T. (1982). Why loneliness occurs: The interrelationship of social-psychological and privacy concepts. In L. A. Peplau, & D. Perlman (Eds.), *Loneliness: A sourcebook of current theory, research and therapy* (pp. 152-165). New York: Wiley.

Diener, E., & Emmons, R. A. (1984). The independence of positive and negative affect. *Journal of Personality and Social Psychology, 47*, 1105-1117.

Dodge, K. A. (1983). Behavioral antecedents of peer social status. *Child Development, 54*, 1386-1399.

Dodge, K. A. (1986). A social information processing model of social competence in children. In M. Perlmutter (Ed.), *Cognitive perspective on children's social and behavioral development* (pp. 77-125). Hillsdale, NJ: Erlbaum.

Dodge, K. A., & Coie, J. D. (1987). Social-information processing factors in reactive and proactive aggression in children's peer groups. *Journal of Personality and Social Psychology, 53*, 1146-1158.

Dodge, K. A., Coie, J. D., & Brakke, N. P. (1982). Behavioral patterns of socially rejected and neglected preadolescents: The role of social approach and aggression. *Journal of Abnormal Child Psychology, 10,* 389-409.

Dumas, J. E. (1986). Parental perception and treatment outcome in families of aggressive children: A causal model. *Behavior Therapy, 17,* 420-432.

Dunst, C. J., Trivette, C. M., & Deal, A. G. (1988). *Enabling and empowering families.* Cambridge, MA: Brookline.

Dyson, L., & Fewell, R. R. (1986). Stress and adaptation in parents of young handicapped children and nonhandicapped children: A comparative study. *Journal of the Division for Early Childhood, 10,* 25-34.

East, P. L. (1991). The parent-child relationships of withdrawn, aggressive and sociable children: Child and parent perspectives. *Merrill-Palmer Quarterly, 37,* 425-443.

Ebata, A., & Moos, R. H. (1991). Coping and adjustment in distressed and healthy adolescents. *Journal of Applied Developmental Psychology, 12,* 33-54.

Eden-Piercy, G. V. S., Blacher, J. B., & Eyman, R. K. (1986). Exploring parents' reactions to their young child with severe handicaps. *Mental Retardation, 24,* 285-291.

Efrati, M. W. (1993). *Family functioning and adolescents' social competence.* Unpublished Master's thesis, Tel Aviv University.

Elliott, S. N., Sheridan, S. M., & Gresham, F. M. (1989). Assessing and treating social skills deficits: A case study for the scientific-practitioner. *Journal of School Psychology, 27,* 197-222.

Ellis, S., Rogoff, B., Cromer, C. C. (1981). Age segregation in children's social interactions. *Developmental Psychology, 17,* 399-407.

Epanchin, B. C., & Rennells, M. S. (1989). Parents' and teachers' sensitivity to unhappiness reported by undercontrolled children. *Behavioral Disorders, 14,* 166-174.

Epstein, M. H., Bursuck, W., & Cullinan, D. (1985). Patterns of behavior problems among the learning disabled: Boys aged 12-18, girls aged 6-11 and girls aged 12-18. *Learning Disability Quarterly, 8,* 123-129.

Erickson, E.H. (1968). *Identity, youth and crisis.* New York: Norton.

Eyberg, S. M. (1992). Assessing therapy outcome with preschool children: Progress and problems. *Journal of Clinical Child Psychology, 21,* 306-311.

Eysenck, H. J., & Eysenck, M. W. (1985). *Personality and individual differences: A natural science approach.* New York: Plenum Press.

Farber, B. (1959). Effects of a severely mentally retarded child on family integration. *Monographs of the Society for Research in Child Development, 24.*

Fessler, M. A., Rosenberg, M. S., & Rosenberg, L. A. (1991). Concomitant learning disabilities and learning problems among students with behavioral/emotional disorders. *Behavioral Disorders, 16,* 97-106.

Florian, V., & Krulik, T. (1991). Loneliness and social support of mothers of chronically ill children. *Social Science and Medicine, 32,* 1291-1296.

Folkman, S., & Lazarus, R. S. (1985). If it changes it must be a process: Study of emotion and coping during three stages of a college examination. *Journal of Personality and Social Psychology, 48,* 150-170.

Folkman, S., & Lazarus, R. S. (1988). Coping as a mediator of emotions. *Journal of Personality and Social Psychology, 54,* 466-475.

Folkman, S., Schaefer, C., & Lazarus, R. S. (1979). Cognitive processes as mediators of stress and coping. In V. Hamilton, & D. M. Warburton (Eds.), *Human stress and cognition: An info-processing approach* (pp. 265-298). London: Wiley.

Forgas, J. P., & Bower, G. H. (1987). Mood effects on person perception judgements. *Journal of Personality and Social Psychology, 53,* 53-60.

Forgas, J. P., Bower, G. H., & Krantz, S. E. (1984). The influence of mood on perceptions of social interactions. *Journal of Experimental Social Psychology, 20,* 497-513.

Forman, S. G. (1980). A comparison of cognitive training and response cost procedures in modifying aggressive behavior of elementary school children. *Behavior Therapy, 11,* 594-600.

Franzoi, S. L., & Davis, M. H. (1985). Adolescent self-disclosure and loneliness: Private self-consciousness and parental influence. *Journal of Personality and Social Psychology, 48,* 768-780.

Fraser, B. C. (1986). Child impairment and parent/infant communication. *Child: Care, Health and Development, 12,* 141-150.

Friedrich, W. N., & Friedrich, W. L. (1981). Psychosocial aspects of parents of handicapped and nonhandicapped children. *American Journal of Mental Deficiency, 85,* 551-553.

Friedrich, W. N., Wilturner, L. T., & Cohen, D. S. (1985). Coping, resources and parenting mentally retarded children. *American Journal of Mental Deficiency, 90,* 130-139.

Fromm-Reichman, F. (1959). Loneliness. *Psychiatry, 22,* 1-15.

Furman, W., & Bierman, K. L. (1984). Children's conceptions of friendship: A multidimensional study of developmental changes. *Developmental Psychology, 20,* 925-931.

Gallagher, J. J., Beckman, P., & Cross, A. H. (1985). Coping resources and parenting mentally retarded children. *American Journal of Mental Deficiency, 90,* 130-139.

Garmezy, N. (1983). Stressors of childhood. In N. Garmezy, & M. Rutter (Eds.) *Stress, coping and development in children* (pp. 43-84). New York: McGraw-Hill Books.

Goldstein, J., Freud, A., & Solnit, A. J. (1979). *Beyond the best interests of the child.* New York: Free Press.

Goldstein, H., & Gallagher, T. M. (1992). Strategies for promoting the social-communicative competence of young children with specific language impairment. In S. L. Odom, S. R. McConnell, & M. A. McEvoy (Eds.), *Social competence of young children with disabilities* (pp. 189-213). Baltimore: Brookes.

Goswick, R. A., & Jones, W. H. (1981). Loneliness, self concept and adjustment. *Journal of Psychology, 107,* 237-240.

Gottman, J., & Fainsilber Katz, L. (1989). The effects of marital discord on young children's peer interaction and health. *Developmental Psychology, 25,* 373-381.

Gottman, J., Gonso, J., & Rasmussen, B. (1975). Social interaction, social competence and friendship in children. *Child Development, 46,* 709-718.

Greenberg, J., & Musham, C. (1981). Avoiding and seeking self-focused attention. *Journal of Research in Personality, 15,* 191-200.

Gresham, F. M. (1981). Assessment of children's social skills. *Journal of School Psychology, 19,* 120-133.

Gresham, F. M. (1986). Conceptual and definitional issues in the assessment of children's social skills: Implications for classification and training. *Journal of Clinical Child Psychology, 15,* 3-15.

Gresham, F. M., & Elliott, S. N. (1984). Assessment and classification of children's social skills: A review of method and issues. *School Psychology Review, 13,* 292-301.

Gresham, F. M., & Elliott, S. N. (1987). The relationship between adaptive behavior and social skills: Issues in definition and assessment. *Journal of Special Education, 21,* 167-181.

Gresham, F. M., & Elliott, S. N. (1990). *Social skills rating system manual.* Circle Pines, MN: American Guidance Service.

Gresham, F. M., & Nagle, R. J. (1980). Social skills training with children: Responsiveness to modeling and coaching as a function of peer orientation. *Journal of Consulting and Clinical Psychology, 48,* 718-729.

Gresham, F. M., & Reschly, D. J. (1986). Social skill deficits and low peer acceptance of mainstreamed learning disabled children. *Learning Disabilities Quarterly, 9,* 23-32.

Guevremont, D. C., MacMillan, V. M., Shawchuck, C. R., & Hansen, D. J. (1989). A peer-mediated intervention with clinic referred socially isolated girls. *Behavior Modification, 13,* 32-50.

Guralnick, M. J. (1992). A hierarchical model for understanding children's peer-related social competence. In S. L. Odom, S. R. McConnell, & M. A. McEvoy (Eds.), *Social competence of young children with disabilities* (pp. 37-64). Baltimore: Brookes.

Guralnick, M. J., & Groom, J. M. (1987). The peer relations of mildly delayed and nonhandicapped preschool children in mainstreamed playgroups. *Child Development, 58,* 1556-1572.

Haddad, J. D., Barocas, R., & Hollenbeck, A. R. (1991). Family organization and parent attitudes of children with conduct disorder. *Journal of Clinical Child Psychology, 20,* 152-161.

Hamre-Nietupski, S., Nietupski, J., & Strathe, M. (1992). Functional life skills, academic skills and friendship/social relationship development: What do parents with moderate/severe/profound disabilities value? *Journal of the Association for Persons with Severe Handicaps, 17,* 53-58.

Hansen, D. J., Watson-Perczel, M. & Christopher, J. S. (1989). Clinical issues in social-skills training with adolescents. *Clinical Psychology Review, 9,* 365-391.

Haring, N. G., & Liberty, K. A. (1990). Matching strategies with performance in facilitating generalization. *Focus on Exceptional Children, 22,* 1-16.

Hart, C., Ladd, G., & Burleson, B. (1990). Children's expectations of the outcomes of social strategies: Relations with sociometric status and maternal disciplinary style. *Child Development, 61,* 127-137.

Hazen, N. L., & Black, B. (1989). Preschool peer communication skills: The role of social status and interaction context. *Child Development, 60,* 867-876.

Hodapp, R. M., Dykens, E. M., Evans, D. W., & Merighi, J. R. (1992). Maternal emotional reactions to young children with different types of handicaps. *Journal of Developmental and Behavioral Pediatrics, 13,* 118-123.

Hofmann, C. (1983). Hausfrauenarbeit und sozialisationsklima in familien von Lerbehinderten sonderschulen. *Behindertenpadagogik, 22,* 226-241.

Hojat, M. (1982a). Loneliness as a function of parent-child and peer relations. *Journal of Psychology, 112,* 129-133.

Hojat, M. (1982b). Loneliness as a function of selected personality variables. *Journal of Clinical Psychology, 38,* 137-141.

Holahan, C. J., & Moos, R. H. (1985). Life stress and health: Personality, coping, and family support in stress resistance. *Journal of Personality and Social Psychology, 47,* 739-747.

Holahan, C. J., & Moos, R. H. (1987a). Personal and contextual determinants of coping strategies. *Journal of Personality and Social Psychology, 52,* 946-955.

Holahan, C. J., & Moos, R. H. (1987b). Risk, resistance and psychological distress: A longitudinal analysis with adults and children. *Journal of Abnormal Psychology, 96,* 3-13.

Holahan, C. J., & Moos, R. H. (1990). Life stressors, resistance factors and improved psychological functioning: An extension of the stress resistance paradigm. *Journal of Personality and Social Psychology, 58,* 909-917.

Hooper, S. R., & Willis, W. G. (1989). *Learning disability subtyping.* New York: Springer-Verlag.

Huesmann, L. R. (1988). An information processing model for the development of aggression. *Aggressive Behavior, 14,* 13-24.

Hughes, J. N., Robinson, M. S., & Moore, L. A. (1991). Children's attributions for peers' positive behaviors: Social status differences. *Journal of Abnormal Child Psychology, 19,* 645-657.

Hundert, J., & Houghton, A. (1992). Promoting social interaction of children with disabilities in integrated preschools: A failure to generalize. *Exceptional Children, 58,* 311-320.

Hymel, S. (1986). Interpretations of peer behavior: Affective bias in childhood and adolescence. *Child Development, 57,* 431-445.

Hymel, S., Frank, S., & Freigang, R. (1985). Peer relationships and their dysfunction: Considering the child's perspective. *Journal of Social and Clinical Psychology, 3,* 405-415.

Hymel, S., Rubin, K. H., Rowden, L., & LeMare, L. (1990). Children's peer relationships: Longitudinal prediction of internalizing and externalizing problems from middle to late childhood. *Child Development, 61,* 2004-2021.

Inderbitzen-Pisaruk, H., Clark, M. L., & Solano, C. H. (1992) Correlates of loneliness in midadolescence. *Journal of Youth and Adolescence, 21,* 151-167.

Iverson, A. M., & Eichler, J. B. (1992, August). *Predicting children's loneliness: Quantity and quality of friendships.* Paper presented at the annual American Psychological Association convention, Washington, DC.

Johnson, D. W., & Johnson, R. T. (1986). Mainstreaming and cooperative learning strategies. *Exceptional Children, 52,* 553-561.

Jolligg, D., & Horne, A. (1986). Social learning family therapy. *Individual Psychology, 42,* 567-582.

Jones, W. H. (1981). Loneliness and social contact. *Journal of Social Psychology, 113,* 295-296.

Jones, W. H. (1982). Loneliness and social behavior. In L. A. Peplau, & D. Perlman (Eds.), *Loneliness: A sourcebook of current theory, research and therapy* (pp. 238-254). New York: Wiley.

Jones, W. H., Freemon, J. A., & Goswick, R. A. (1981). The persistence of loneliness: Self and other determinants. *Journal of Personality, 49,* 27-48.

Jones, W. H., Hobbs, S. A., & Hockenberry, D. (1982). Loneliness and social skill deficits. *Journal of Personality and Social Psychology, 42,* 682-689.

Josselson, R. (1992). *The space between us.* San Francisco: Jossey-Bass.

Jupp, J. J., & Griffiths, M. D. (1990). Self-concept changes in shy, socially isolated adolescents following social skills training emphasizing role plays. *Australian Psychologist, 25,* 165-177.

Juvonen, J. (1991, April). *The effect of attributions and interpersonal attitudes on social emotions and behavior.* Paper presented at the annual American Educational Research Association conference, Chicago.

Kalliopuska, M., & Laitinen, M. (1991). Loneliness related to self-concept. *Psychological Reports, 69,* 27-34.

Kavale, K. A., & Forness, S. R. (1992). History, definition, and diagnosis. In N. N. Singh, & I. L. Beale (Eds.), *Learning disabilities: Nature, theory and treatment* (pp. 3-43). New York: Springer-Verlag.

Kazak, A. E. (1987). Families with disabled children: Stress and social networks in three samples. *Journal of Abnormal Child Psychology, 15,* 137-146.

Kazak, A. F., & Marvin, R. S. (1984). Differences, difficulties, and adaptation: Stress and social networks in families with a handicapped child. *Family Relations, 33,* 67-77.

Kazdin, A. E. (1987). *Conduct disorders in childhood and adolescence.* Newbury Park, CA: Sage.

Keltikangas-Jarvinen, L., & Kangas, P. (1988). Problem-solving strategies in aggressive and nonaggressive children. *Aggressive Behavior, 14,* 255-264.

Kobasa, S. C. (1982). Commitment and coping in stress resistance among lawyers. *Journal of Personality and Social Psychology, 42,* 707-717.

Kohler, F. W., Schwartz, I. S., Cross, J. A., & Fowler, S. P. (1989). The effect of two alternating peer intervention roles on independent work skills. *Education and Treatment of Children, 12,* 205-218.

Kopp, C. B., Baker, B. L., & Brown, K. W. (1992). Social skills and their correlates: Preschoolers with developmental delays. *American Journal on Mental Retardation, 26,* 357-366.

Kupersmidt, J. B., Coie, J. D., & Dodge, K. A. (1990). The role of poor peer relations in the development of disorder. In S. R. Asher, & J. D. Coie (Eds.), *Peer rejection in childhood* (pp. 274-305). Cambridge, England: University Press.

Ladd, G. W. (1981). Effectiveness of a social learning method for enhancing children's social interaction and peer acceptance. *Child Development, 52,* 171-178.

Ladd, G. W. (1983). Social networks of popular, average and rejected children in school settings. *Merrill-Palmer Quarterly, 29,* 283-307.

Ladd, G. W. (1988). Friendship patterns and peer status during early and middle childhood. *Developmental and Behavioral Pediatrics, 9,* 229-238.

Ladd, G. W., & Asher, S. R. (1985). Social skill training and children's peer relations. In L. L'Abate, & M. Milan (Eds.),

Handbook of social skills training (pp. 219-244). New York: Wiley.

Ladd, G. W., & Emerson, E. S. (1984). Shared knowledge in children's friendships. *Developmental Psychology, 20,* 932-940.

Ladd, G. W., Hart, C. H., & Wadsworth, E. M. (1988). Preschoolers' peer networks in nonschool settings: Relationships to family characteristics and school adjustment. In J. Antrobus, M. Hammer, & S. Salzinger (Eds.), *Social networks of children, adolescents and college students* (pp. 61-92). New York: Erlbaum.

LaFreniere, P., & Sroufe, L. A. (1985). Profiles of peer competence in the preschool: Interrelations between measures, influence of social ecology, and relation to attachment history. *Developmental Psychology, 21,* 46-49.

LaGreca, A. M., & Santogrossi, D. (1980). Social skills training with elementary school students: A behavioral group approach. *Journal of Consulting and Clinical Psychology, 48,* 220-227.

Lancioni, G. E. (1982). Normal children as tutors to teach social responses to withdrawn mentally retarded schoolmates: Training, maintenance and generalization. *Journal of Applied Behavior Analysis, 15,* 17-40.

Landau, S., & Milich, R. (1985). Social status of aggressive and aggressive/withdrawn boys: A replication across age and method. *Journal of Consulting and Clinical Psychology, 53,* 141.

Large, T. (1989). Some aspects of loneliness in families. *Family Process, 28,* 23-35.

Lazarus, R. S., & Folkman, S. (1984). *Stress, appraisal, and coping.* New York: Springer-Verlag.

Ledingham, J. E. (1981). Developmental patterns of aggressive and withdrawn behaviors in childhood: A possible method for identifying preschizophrenics. *Journal of Abnormal Child Psychology, 9,* 1-22.

Ledingham, J. E., & Schwartzman, A. F. (1984). A 3-year follow-up of aggressive and withdrawn behavior in childhood: Preliminary findings. *Journal of Abnormal Child Psychology, 12,* 157-168.

Litt, M. D. (1988). Cognitive mediators of stressful experience: Self-efficacy and perceived control. *Cognitive Therapy and Research, 12,* 241-260.

Lobdell, J., & Perman, D. (1986). The intergeneration transmission of loneliness: A study of college females and their parents. *Journal of Marriage and the Family, 48,* 489-495.

Lochman, J. E. (1985). Effects of different treatment lengths in cognitive behavioral interventions with aggressive boys. *Child Psychiatry and Human Development, 16,* 45-56.

Lochman, J. E. (1988, September). *Long-term efficacy of cognitive behavioral interventions with aggressive boys.* Paper presented at the World Congress on Behavior Therapy, Edinburgh.

Lochman, J. E., Bruch, P. R., & Curry, J. F., & Lampron, L. B. (1984). Treatment and generalization effects of cognitive-behavioral and goal-setting interventions with aggressive boys. *Journal of Counseling and Clinical Psychology, 52,* 915-916.

Lochman, J. E., Lampron, L. B., Bruch, P. R., & Curry, J. F. (1985). Client characteristics associated with behavior change for treated and untreated aggressive boys. *Journal of Abnormal Child Psychology, 13,* 527-538.

Loney, J., & Milich, R. (1982). Hyperactivity, inattention and aggression in clinical practice. In M. Wolraich, & D. Routh (Eds.), *Advances in developmental and behavioral pediatrics* (Vol. 2, pp. 113-147). Greenwich, CT: JAI Press.

Luftig, R. L. (1987). Children's loneliness, perceived ease in making friends and estimated social adequacy: Development and social metacognition. *Child Study Journal, 17,* 35-53.

Luftig, R. L. (1988). Assessment of the perceived school loneliness and isolation of mentally retarded and nonretarded students. *American Journal of Mental Retardation, 92,* 472-475.

Lunt, P. K. (1991). The perceived causal structure of loneliness. *Journal of Personality and Social Psychology, 61,* 26-34.

Maccoby, E. E. (1990). Gender and relationships: A developmental perspective. *American Psychologist, 45,* 513-520.

Maccoby, E. E., & Jacklin, C. (1980). Sex differences in aggression: A rejoinder and reprise. *Child Development, 51,* 964-980.

Maccoby, E. E., & Martin, J. (1983). Socialization in the context of the family: Parent-child interactions. In E. M. Hertherington (Ed.), *Handbook of child psychology: Socialization, personality and social development* (Vol. 4, 4th ed., pp. 1-101). New York: Wiley.

Mahler, M., Pine F., & Bergman, A. (1975). *The psychological birth of the human infant.* New York: Basic Books.

Mahoney, M. J. (1991). *Human change processes.* New York: Basic Books.

Malekoff, A., & Kolodny, R. L. (1991). Memories and memory building: Reflections on group work with the lonely child. *Social Work with Groups, 14,* 87-103.

Marcoen, A., & Goossens, L. (1990, April). *Loneliness and aloneness in adolescence: Introducing a multidimensional measure and some developmental perspectives.* Paper presented at the annual American Educational Research Association conference, Boston.

Margalit, M. (1984). Leisure activities of learning disabled children as a reflection of their passive life style and prolonged dependency. *Child Psychiatry and Human Development, 15,* 133-141.

Margalit, M. (1985). Perceptions of parents' behavior, familial satisfaction, and sense of coherence in hyperactive children. *Journal of School Psychology, 23,* 355-364.

Margalit, M. (1988). Introversion/extraversion perspectives in the subgrouping of conduct disorders in Israel. In D. H. Saklofske, & S. B. G. Eysenck (Eds.), *Individual differences in children and adolescents: International perspectives* (pp. 99-107). London: Hodder and Stoughton.

Margalit, M. (1989). Academic competence and social adjustment of boys with learning disabilities and boys with behavior disorders. *Journal of Learning Disabilities, 22,* 41-45.

Margalit, M. (1990a). *Effective technology integration for disabled children: The family perspective.* New York: Springer-Verlag.

Margalit, M. (1990b, July). *Fostering the sense of coherence among children with special needs and their parents.* Paper presented at the Children in War Conference, Jerusalem, Israel.

Margalit, M. (1991a, October). *Feelings of loneliness in students with learning disabilities.* Paper presented at the annual International Academy of Research in Learning Disabilities conference, Cincinnati.

Margalit, M. (1991b). Promoting classroom adjustment and social skills for students with mental retardation within an experimental and control group design. *Exceptionality, 2,* 195-204.

Margalit, M. (1991c). Understanding loneliness among students with learning disabilities. *Behavior Change, 8,* 167-173.

Margalit, M. (1992). *Subtypes of family functioning as related to adolescents' social adjustment and loneliness.* Unpublished manuscript, Tel Aviv University.

Margalit, M. (1993a). *Social competence and loneliness among three groups of special education students.* Manuscript in preparation, Tel Aviv University.

Margalit, M. (1993b, October). *Social adjustment of behaviorally disordered and learning disabled students.* Paper presented at the Council of Learning Disabilities annual meeting, Baltimore.

Margalit, M. (in press). Social skills and classroom behavior among adolescents with mild mental retardation. *American Journal of Mental Retardation.*

Margalit, M., & Al-Yagon, M. (in press). Learning disability subtyping, loneliness, and classroom adjustment. *Learning Disability Quarterly.*

Margalit, M., & Ankonina, D. B. (1991). Positive and negative affect in parenting disabled children. *Counseling Psychology Quarterly, 4,* 289-299.

Margalit, M., & Ben-Dov, I. (1992, March). *Kibbutz versus city comparisons of social competence and loneliness among students with and without learning disabilities.* Paper presented at the annual International Academy of Research in Learning Disabilities conference, Amsterdam.

Margalit, M., & Heiman, T. (1984, October). *Family climate and anxiety expressions of families with a learning disabled boy.* Paper presented at the annual Council of Learning Disabilities conference, Dallas.

Margalit, M., & Heiman, T. (1986). Learning disabled boys' anxiety, parental anxiety, and family climate. *Journal of Clinical Child Psychology, 15,* 248-253.

Margalit, M., Leyser, Y., Ankonina, D. B., & Avraham, Y. (1991). Community support in Israeli kibbutz and city families of disabled children: Family climate and parental coherence. *Journal of Special Education, 24,* 427-440.

Margalit, M., Leyser, Y., Avraham, Y., & Lewy-Osin, M. (1988). Social-environmental characteristics (family climate) and sense of coherence in kibbutz families with disabled and non-disabled children. *European Journal of Special Needs Education, 3,* 87-98.

Margalit, M., & Raviv, A. (1983). Mothers' perceptions of the family climate in families of retarded children. *Exceptional Child, 30,* 163-169.

Margalit, M., Raviv, A., & Ankonina, D. B. (1992). Coping and coherence among parents with disabled children. *Journal of Clinical Child Psychology, 21,* 202-209.

Margalit, M., Raviv, A., & Pahn-Steinmetz, N. (1988). Social competence of learning disabled children: Cognitive and emotional aspects. *Exceptional Child, 35,* 179-189.

Margalit, M., & Ronen, T. (1993). Loneliness and social competence among preadolescents and adolescents with mild mental retardation. *Mental Handicap Research, 6,* 97-111.

Margalit, M., & Zak, I. (1984). Anxiety and self-concept of learning disabled children. *Journal of Learning Disabilities, 17,* 537-539.

Masters, J. C., & Furman, W. (1981). Popularity, individual friendship selection, and specific peer interaction among children. *Developmental Psychology, 17,* 344-350.

McCubbin, H. I., & Patterson, J. M. (1983). The family stress process: The double ABCX model of adjustment and adaptation. *Journal of Marriage Family Review, 6,* 7-37.

McEvoy, M. A., Odom, S. L., & McConnell. S. R. (1992). Peer social competence intervention for young children with disabilities. In S. L. Odom, S. R. McConnell, & M. A. McEvoy (Eds.), *Social competence of young children with disabilities* (pp. 113-133). Baltimore: Brookes.

McGee, R., Williams, S., & Silva, P. A. (1984). Background characteristics of aggressive, hyperactive and aggressive/hyperactive boys. *Journal of the American Academy of Child Psychiatry, 23,* 280-284.

McKinney, J. D. (1988). Research on conceptually and empirically derived subtypes of specific learning disabilities. In M. D. Wang, H. J. Waller, & M. C. Reynolds (Eds.), *The handbook of special education: Research and practice* (pp. 253-281). Oxford, England: Pergamon.

Medora, N., & Woodward, J. C. (1986). Loneliness among adolescent college students at a midwestern university. *Adolescence, 21,* 391-402.

Mikulincer, M., & Segal, J. (1991). Loneliness and the desire for intimacy: The intervening role of locus of control. *Personality and Individual Differences, 12,* 801-809.

Milich, R., & Landau, S. (1984). A comparison of the social status and social behavior of aggressive and aggressive/withdrawn boys. *Journal of Abnormal Child Psychology, 12,* 277-288.

Mize, J., & Ladd, G. W. (1990). Toward the development of successful social skills training for preschool children. In S. R. Asher, & J. D. Coie (Eds.), *Peer rejection in childhood* (pp. 338-361). Cambridge, England: University Press.

Moore, D., & Schultz, N. R. (1983). Loneliness at adolescence: Correlates, attributions and coping. *Journal of Youth and Adolescence, 12,* 95-100.

Moos, R. H. (1987). Learning environments in context: Links between school, work and family settings. In B. J. Fraser (Ed.), *The study of learning environments* (Vol. 2, pp. 1-16). Perth, Australia: Curtin University of Technology.

Moos, R.H. (1991). Connections between school, work and family settings. In B. J. Fraser, & H. J. Walberg (Eds.), *Educational environments: Evaluation, antecedents and consequences* (pp. 29-53). Oxford, England: Pergamon.

Moos, R. H., Cronkite, R. C., Billings, A. G., & Finney, J. W. (1987). *Revised health and daily living form manual.* Veterans Administration and Stanford University Medical Centers, Palo Alto, CA.

Moos, R. H., & Moos, B. S. (1976). A typology of family social environments. *Family Process, 15,* 357-371.

Moos, R. H., & Moos, B. S. (1983). Adaptation and the quality of life in work and family settings. *Journal of Community Psychology, 11,* 158-170.

Moos, R. H., & Moos, B. S. (1986). *Family environment scale manual* (2nd ed.). Palo Alto, CA: Consulting Psychologists Press.

Mullins, J. B. (1987). Authentic voices from parents of exceptional children. *Family Relations, 36,* 30-33.

Murphy, J. S., & Newlon, B. J. (1987). Loneliness in the mainstreamed hearing impaired college student. *American Annals of the Deaf, 132,* 21-25,

Nelson, G. (1984). The relationship between dimensions of classroom and family environments and the self-concept, satisfaction, and achievement of grade 7 and 8 students. *Journal of Community Psychology, 12,* 276-287.

Nimi, A., Uemura, K. (1987). Stresses on the parents of a handicapped child in school age: Analysis of stress patterns and descriptions of representative mothers' stress. *Japanese Journal of Special Education, 25,* 29-38.

Oden, S. L., & Asher, S. R. (1977). Coaching children in social skills for friendship making. *Child Development, 48,* 495-506.

Odom, S. L., McConnell, S. R., & McEvoy, M. A. (1992). Peer-related social competence and its significance for young children with disabilities. In S. L. Odom, S. R. McConnell, & M. A. McEvoy (Eds.), *Social competence of young children with disabilities* (pp. 3-35). Baltimore: Brookes.

Olson, D. H. (1986). Circumplex model VII: Validation studies and FACES III. *Family Process, 25,* 337-351.

Overholser, J. C. (1992). Interpersonal dependency and social loss. *Personality and Individual Differences, 13,* 17-23.

Ozer, E. M., & Bandura, A. (1990). Mechanisms governing empowerment effects: A self-efficacy analysis. *Journal of Personality and Social Psychology, 58,* 472-486.

Page, R. M. (1991a). Assisting children to avoid loneliness and isolation. *Journal of Instructional Psychology, 18,* 69-72.

Page, R. M. (1991b). Loneliness as a risk factor in adolescent hopelessness. *Journal of Research in Personality, 25,* 189-195.

Panella, D., & Henggeler, S. W. (1986). Peer interactions of conduct-disordered, anxious-withdrawn, and well-adjusted black adolescents. *Journal of Abnormal Child Psychology, 14,* 1-11.

Paris, S. G., & Oka, E. R. (1989). Strategies for comprehending text and coping with reading difficulties. *Learning Disabilities Quarterly, 12,* 32-42.

Parker, J. G., & Asher, S. R. (1987). Peer relations and later personal adjustment: Are low-accepted children "at risk?" *Psychological Bulletin, 102,* 357-389.

Parker, J. G., & Asher, S. R. (in press). Friendship and friendship quality in middle childhood: Links with peer group acceptance and feelings of loneliness and social dissatisfaction. *Developmental Psychology.*

Parkhurst, J. T., & Asher, S. R. (1992). Peer rejection in middle school: Subgroup differences in behavior, loneliness and interpersonal concern. *Developmental Psychology, 28,* 231-241.

Patterson, G. R. (1980). Mothers: The unacknowledged victims. *Monographs of the Society for Research in Child Development, 45* (5, serial 186).

Patterson, G. R. (1982). *Coercive family process.* Eugene, OR: Castalia.

Patterson, G. R., & Reid, J. B. (1984). Social interactional processes in the family: The study of moment to moment family transactions in which human social development is embedded. *Journal of Applied Developmental Psychology, 5,* 237-262.

Pearl, R. (1992). Psychosocial characteristics of learning disabled students. In N. N. Singh, & I. A. Beale (Eds.), *Learning disabilities: Nature, theory and treatment* (pp. 96-125). New York: Springer-Verlag.

Pellegrini, D. S., & Urbain, E. S. (1985). An evaluation of the interpersonal cognitive problem solving training with children. *Journal of Child Psychology and Psychiatry, 26,* 17-41.

Peplau, L. A., Miceli, M., & Morasch, B. (1982). Loneliness and self-evaluation. In L. A. Peplau, & D. Perlman (Eds.), *Loneliness: A sourcebook of current theory, research and therapy* (pp. 135-151). New York: Wiley.

Peplau, L. A., & Perlman, D. (1982). Perspectives on loneliness. In L. A. Peplau, & D. Perlman (Eds.), *Loneliness: A sourcebook of current theory, research and therapy* (pp. 1-18). New York: Wiley.

Perlman, D., & Peplau, L. A. (1982). Theoretical approaches to loneliness. In L. A. Peplau, & D. Perlman (Eds.), *Loneliness: A sourcebook of current theory, research and therapy* (pp. 123-134). New York: Wiley.

Perlmutter, B. F., Crocker, J., Cordray, D., & Garstecki, D. (1983). Sociometric status and related personality characteristics of mainstreamed learning disabled adolescents. *Learning Disabilities Quarterly, 6,* 20-30.

Petersen, A. C. (1988). Adolescent development. *Annual Review of Psychology, 39,* 593-607.

Pettit, G., Dodge, K., & Brown, M. (1988). Early family experience, social problem solving patterns, and children's social competence. *Child Development, 59,* 107-120.

Plienis, A. J., Hansen, D. J., Ford, F., & Smith, S. (1987). Behavioral small group training to improve the social skills of emotionally disordered adolescents. *Behavior Therapy, 18,* 17-32.

Prage, M. E., Greenbaum, P. E., & Friedman, R. M. (1992, August). *Predictive utility of aggressive versus non-aggressive subtyping of adolescents with conduct disorder behaviors.* Paper presented at the annual American Psychological Association convention, Washington, DC.

Prage, M. E., Greenbaum, P. E., Silver, S. E., Friedman, R. M., Kutash, K., & Duchnowski, A. J. (1992). Family functioning and psychopathology among adolescents with severe emotional disturbances. *Journal of Abnormal Child Psychology, 20*, 83-102.

Putallaz, M., & Hope-Heflin, A. (1990). Parent-child interaction. In S. R. Asher, & J. D. Coie (Eds.), *Peer rejection in childhood* (pp. 189-216). Cambridge, England: University Press.

Putallaz, M., & Wasserman, A. (1990). Children's entry behavior. In S. R. Asher, & J. D. Coie (Eds.), *Peer rejection in childhood* (pp. 60-89). Cambridge, England: University Press.

Quay, H. C. (1983). A dimensional approach to behavior disorders: A revised behavior problem checklist. *School Psychological Review, 12*, 244-249.

Rizzo, T. A. (1988). The relationship between friendship and sociometric judgements of peer acceptance and rejection. *Child Study Journal, 18*, 161-191.

Rodger, S. (1987). A comparison between parenting a normal and a handicapped child throughout the lifespan. *British Journal of Occupational Therapy, 50*, 167-170.

Rogers, H., & Saklofske, D. H. (1985). Self concept, locus of control, and performance expectations of learning disabled children. *Journal of Learning Disabilities, 18*, 273-287.

Rook, K. S. (1984). Promoting social bonding. *American Psychologist, 39*, 1389-1407.

Rook, K, S., & Peplau, L. A. (1982). Perspectives on helping the lonely. In L. A. Peplau, & D. Perlman (Eds.), *Loneliness: A sourcebook of current theory, research and therapy* (pp. 351-378). New York: Wiley.

Roth, S., & Cohen, L. J. (1986). Approach, avoidance and coping with stress. *American Psychologist, 41*, 813-819.

Rothbart, M. (1986). Longitudinal observation of infant temperament. *Developmental Psychology, 22*, 356-365.

Rothbaum, F., & Weisz, J. R. (1989). *Child psychopathology and the quest for control*. Newbury Park, CA: Sage.

Rubenstein, C., & Shaver, P. (1980). Loneliness in two northeastern cities. In J. Hartog, J. R. Audy, & Y. A. Cohen (Eds.), *The anatomy of loneliness* (pp. 319-337). New York: International Universities Press.

Rubin, K. H. (1985). Socially withdrawn children: An "at risk" population? In B. H. Schneider, K. H. Rubin, & J. E. Ledingham (Eds.), *Peer relationships and social skills in childhood: Issues in assessment and training* (pp.125-139). New York: Springer-Verlag.

Rubin, K. H., & Clark, M. L. (1983). Preschool teachers' ratings of behavioral problems: Observational, sociometric and social-cognitive correlates. *Journal of Abnormal Child Psychology, 11,* 273-285.

Rubin, K. H., & Daniels-Beirness, T. (1983). Concurrent and predictive correlates of sociometric status in kindergarten and grade 1 children. *Merrill-Palmer Quarterly, 29,* 337-351.

Rubin, K. H., LeMare, L. J., & Lollis, S. (1990). Social withdrawal in childhood: Developmental pathways to peer rejection. In S. R. Asher, & J. D. Coie (Eds.), *Peer rejection in childhood* (pp. 219-249). Cambridge, England: University Press.

Rubin, K. H., & Mills, R. S. L. (1988). The many faces of social isolation in childhood. *Journal of Consulting and Clinical Psychology, 56,* 916-924.

Rubin, Z., & Slomon, J. (1984). How parents influence their children's friendships. In M. Lewis (Ed.), *Beyond the dyad* (pp. 223-250). New York: Plenum Press.

Russell, D., Cutrona, C. E., Rose, J., & Yurko, K. (1984). Social and emotional loneliness: An examination of Weiss' typology of loneliness. *Journal of Personality and Social Psychology, 46,* 1313-1321.

Ryan, R. M., & Powelson, C. L. (1991, April). *Autonomy and relatedness as fundamental to motivation in education.* Paper presented at the annual American Educational Research Association conference, Chicago.

Ryde-Brandt, B. (1990). Anxiety and defence strategies in mothers of children with different disabilities. *British Journal of Medical Psychology, 63,* 183-192.

Sabornie, E. J., & Kauffman, J. M. (1986). Social acceptance of learning disabled adolescents. *Learning Disabilities Quarterly, 9,* 55-60.

Sabornie, E. J., Kauffman, J. M., Ellis, E. S., Marshall, K. J., & Elksnin, L. K. (1987-1988). Bi-directional and cross-categorical social status of LD, BD, and nonhandicapped adolescents. *Journal of Special Education, 21,* 39-56.

Sabornie, E. J., Marshall, K. J., & Ellis, E. S. (1988, April). *Received and assigned regular classroom social status of students with learning disabilities and behavior disorders.* Paper presented at the annual American Educational Research Association conference, New Orleans, LA.

Sabornie, E. J., & Thomas, V. (1989, April). *Social/affective adjustment of mildly handicapped and nonhandicapped early adolescents.* Paper presented at the annual American Educational Research Association conference, San Francisco.

Schneider, M. J., & Leitenberg, H. (1989). A comparison of aggressive and withdrawn children's self-esteem, optimism and pessimism and causal attributions for success and failure. *Journal of Abnormal Child Psychology, 17,* 133-144.

Schunk, D. H., & Hanson, A. R. (1985). Peer models: Influence on children's self-efficacy and achievement. *Journal of Educational Psychology, 77,* 313-322.

Schunk, D. H., Hanson, A. R., & Cox, P. D. (1987). Peer-model attributes and children's achievement behavior. *Journal of Educational Psychology, 79,* 54-61.

Seigel, L. S., & Metsala, J. (1992). An alternative to the food processor approach to subtypes of learning disabilities. In N. N. Singh, & I. L. Beale (Eds.), *Learning disabilities: Nature, theory and treatment* (pp. 44-60). New York: Springer-Verlag.

Seligman, M., & Darling, R. B. (1989). *Ordinary families, special children.* New York: Guilford Press.

Sheeber, L. B., & Johnson, J. H.(1992). Child temperament, maternal adjustment and changes in family life style. *American Journal of Orthopsychiatry, 62,* 178-185.

Short, E. J., Schatschneider, C. W., & Friebert, S. E. (1992). Inactive learner hypothesis: Myth or reality. In N. N. Singh, & I. L. Beale (Eds.), *Learning disabilities: Nature, theory and treatment* (pp. 302-326). New York: Springer-Verlag.

Shure, M. B., & Spivack, G. (1978). *Problem-solving techniques in child-rearing.* San Francisco: Jossey-Bass.

Shure, M. B., & Spivack, G. (1979). Interpersonal cognitive problem solving and primary prevention: Programming for preschool and kindergarten children. *Journal of Clinical Child Psychology, 2,* 89-94.

Siegel, L. S., & Cunningham, C. E. (1984). Social interactions: A transactional approach with illustrations from children with developmental problems. In A. Doyle, D. Gold, & D. S. Moskowitz (Eds.), *Children in families under stress* (pp. 85-98). San Francisco: Jossey-Bass.

Solano, C. H., Batten. P. G., & Parish, E. A. (1982). Loneliness and patterns of self-disclosure. *Journal of Personality and Social Psychology, 43,* 524-531.

Solnit, A. J. (March, 1986). *Children's rights and needs in the light of new research.* Paper presented as the first Milton and Eleanor Former Lecture On Early Childhood Education, Hebrew University, Jerusalem.

Solomon, Z., Mikulincer, M., & Avitzur, E. (1988). Coping, locus of control, social support, and combat-related post-traumatic stress disorder: A prospective study. *Journal of Personality and Social Psychology, 55,* 279-285.

Spitzberg, B. H., & Hurt, T. H. (1987). The relationship of interpersonal competence and skills to reported loneliness across time. *Journal of Social Behavior and Personality, 2,* 157-172.

Stern, D. (1985). *The interpersonal world of the infant.* New York: Basic Books.

Stone, W. L., & LaGreca, A. M. (1990). The social status of children with learning disabilities: A reexamination. *Journal of Learning Disabilities, 23,* 32-37.

Storr, A. (1988). *Solitude.* New York: Ballantine.

Sullivan, H.S. (1953). *The interpersonal theory of psychiatry.* New York: Norton.

Swanson, H. L. (1990). Instruction derived from the strategy deficit model: Overview of principles and procedures. In T. E. Scruggs & B. Y. L. Wong (Eds.), *Intervention research on learning disabilities* (pp. 34-65). New York: Springer-Verlag.

Taylor, A. R., Asher, S. R., & Williams, G. A. (1987). The social adaptation of mainstreamed mildly retarded children. *Child Development, 58,* 1321-1334.

Tiggemann, M., Winefield, A. H., Winefield, H. R., & Goldney, R. D. (1991). The stability of attributional style and its relation to psychological distress. *British Journal of Clinical Psychology, 30,* 247-255.

Trivette, C. M., Dunst, C. J., Deal, A. G., Hamer, A. W., & Propst, S. (1990). Assessing family strengths and family functioning style. *Topics in Early Childhood Special Education, 10,* 16-35.

Turnbull, A. P., & Turnbull, H. R. (1986). *Families, professionals and exceptionality.* Columbus, OH: Merrill.

Twardosz, S., Nordquist, V. M., Simon, R., & Botkin, D. (1983). The effect of group affection activities on the interaction of socially isolated children. *Analysis and Intervention in Developmental Disabilities, 13,* 311-338.

Unger, Y. (1992). *Social competence and feelings of loneliness among adolescents with learning disabilities: Self-reports and mothers' and teachers' ratings.* Unpublished Master's thesis, Tel Aviv University.

Van-Buskirk, A. M., & Duke, M. P. (1991). The relationship between coping style and loneliness in adolescents: Can "sad passivity" be adaptive? *Journal of Genetic Psychology, 152,* 145-157.

Vaughn, S., & Hogan, A. (1990). Social competence and learning disabilities: A prospective study. In H. L. Swanson, & B. Keogh (Eds.), *Learning disabilities: Theoretical and research issues* (pp. 175-191). Hillsdale, NJ: Erlbaum.

Vaughn, S., Hogan, A., Kouzekanani, K., & Shapiro, S. (1990). Peer acceptance, self perceptions, and social skills of learning disabled students prior to identification. *Journal of Educational Psychology, 82,* 101-106.

Vaughn, S., & LaGreca, A. M. (1992). Beyond greetings and making friends: Social skills from a broader perspective. In B. Y. L. Wong (Ed.), *Contemporary intervention research in learning disabilities: An international perspective* (pp. 96-114). New York: Springer-Verlag.

Vaughn, S., McIntosh, R., & Hogan, A. (1990). Why social skills training doesn't work: An alternative model. In T. E. Scruggs, & B. Y. L. Wong (Eds.), *Intervention research on learning disabilities* (pp. 279-303). New York: Springer-Verlag.

Vaux, A. (1987). Appraisals of social support: Love, respect and involvement. *Journal of Community Psychology, 15,* 493-502.

Vitkus, J., & Horowitz, L. M. (1987). Poor social performance of lonely people: Lacking a skill or adopting a role. *Journal of Personality and Social Psychology, 52,* 1266-1273.

Vuchinich, S., Bank, L., & Patterson, G. R. (1992). Parenting, peers and the stability of antisocial behavior in preadolescent boys. *Developmental Psychology, 28,* 610-521.

Waas, G. A., & Honer, S. A. (1990). Situational attributions and dispositional inferences: The development of peer reputation. *Merrill-Palmer Quarterly, 36,* 239-260.

Walberg, H. J., & Tsai, S. L. (1983). Matthew effects in education. *American Educational Research Journal, 20,* 359-373.

Wallander, J. L., Varni, J. W., Babani, L., Banis, H. T., & Wilcox, K. T. (1988). Children with chronic physical disorders: Maternal reports of their psychological adjustment. *Journal of Pediatric Psychology, 13,* 197-212.

Wasik, B. H. (1987). Sociometric measures and peer descriptions of kindergarten children: A study of reliability and validity. *Journal of Clinical Child Psychology, 16,* 218-224.

Weiner, B. (1985). An attributional theory of achievement motivation and emotion. *Psychological Review, 92,* 548-573.

Weiner, B., & Handel, S. J. (1985). A cognition-emotion-action sequence: Anticipated emotional consequences of causal attributions and reported communication strategy. *Developmental Psychology, 21,* 102-107.

Weiss, R. S. (1973). *Loneliness: The experience of emotional and social isolation.* Cambridge, MA: MIT Press.

Weiss, R. S. (1974). The provisions of social relationships. In Z. Rubin (Ed.), *Doing unto others* (pp. 17-26). Englewood Cliffs, NJ: Prentice-Hall.

Weiss, R. S. (1982). Issues in the study of loneliness. In L. A. Peplau, & D. Perlman (Eds.), *Loneliness: A sourcebook of current theory, research and therapy* (pp. 71-80). New York: Wiley.

Weiss, R. S. (1987). Reflections on the present state of loneliness research. Special Issue: Loneliness: Theory, research and applications. *Journal of Social Behavior and Personality, 2,* 1-16.

Wheeler, V. A., & Ladd, G. W. (1982). Assessment of children's self-efficacy for social interactions with peers. *Developmental Psychology, 18,* 795-805.

Widerstrom, A. H., & Dudley-Marling, C. (1986). Living with a handicapped child: Myth and reality. *Childhood Education, 62,* 359-367.

Williams, G. A., & Asher, S. R. (1990, April). *Loneliness among mildly mentally retarded and nonretarded children in elementary school.* Paper presented at the American Educational Research Association conference, Boston.

Williams, G. A., & Asher, S. R. (1992). Assessment of loneliness at school among children with mild mental retardation. *American Journal of Mental Retardation, 96,* 373-385.

Wilton, K., & Renault, J. (1986). Stress levels in families with intellectually handicapped preschool children and families with nonhandicapped preschool children. *Journal of Mental Deficiency Research, 30,* 163-169.

Winnicott, D. W. (1965). The capacity to be alone. In D. W. Winnicott (Ed.), *The maturation processes and the facilitating environment* (pp. 29-36). New York: International Universities Press.

Woodward, H. (1988). *The solitude of loneliness.* Lexington, MA: Lexington Books.

Woodward, J. C., & Kalyan-Masih, V. (1990). Loneliness, coping strategies and cognitive styles of the gifted rural adolescent. *Adolescence, 25,* 977-988.

Young, E. F. (1982). Loneliness, depression and cognitive therapy: Theory and application. In L. A. Peplau, & D. Perlman (Eds.), *Loneliness: A sourcebook of current theory, research and therapy* (pp. 379-405). New York: Wiley.

Zehavi, I. (1992). *Comparison between students with learning disabilities and nondisabled students on social competence and feelings of loneliness: A developmental perspective.* Unpublished Master's thesis, Tel Aviv University.

Author Index

Subject Index

MIX
Papier aus verantwortungsvollen Quellen
Paper from responsible sources
FSC® C105338

If you have any concerns about our products,
you can contact us on
ProductSafety@springernature.com

In case Publisher is established outside the EU,
the EU authorized representative is:
Springer Nature Customer Service Center GmbH
Europaplatz 3, 69115 Heidelberg, Germany

Printed by Libri Plureos GmbH
in Hamburg, Germany